Praise for
Claiming the Corner Office

"Distilled from the experiences of the authors and other successful leaders, this lively volume is a thoughtful and energetic foray into the foundations of successful leadership. Curran and Fitzpatrick have provided us with a very welcome addition to both the nursing literature and the more general discourse on what it takes to be an effective leader."

–Harold T. Shapiro, PhD
President Emeritus and Professor of Economics and Public Affairs
Princeton University

"*Claiming the Corner Office* is unquestionably a book that is not restricted to the nursing field. Curran and Fitzpatrick have unveiled the balance of tradition and innovation in this engaging and inspiring publication. Many say they aspire to be a leader, but many fall short, characteristically due to lack of knowledge and motivation. Not only have these two successful ladies achieved the 'corner office,' but they've also generously shared the perfect road map for those who have the passion and desire to make the journey. After reading this book, you have no more excuses. You would do your colleagues and friends a disservice by not sharing the invaluable gems that are nestled between the covers of this publication."

–Alan Tanielian
CEO, AlanTown Investments, LLC

"*Claiming the Corner Office* is practical and easy to read— a pitch-perfect guide for nurse practitioners looking for some help in breaking into a C-suite job. The book also is academically sound and calls out the macro trends in health care that put nurse practitioners at the center of what will clearly be some new and important business opportunities. Kudos to Curran and Fitzpatrick."

–Brad Wechsler
Co-Chairman, Assay Healthcare Solutions; Chairman, IMAX Corporation
NYU Langone Medical Center

"Curran and Fitzpatrick have produced a 'must-read' for anyone, especially a nurse whose professional goal is to claim the corner office. The book contains valuable insights, stories, and various experiences that will prove to be immensely helpful to the reader."

–*Jim Skogsbergh, MHA, FACHE*
President and CEO, Advocate Health Care

"This book is filled with practical wisdom, backed up by academic rigor. If you are not sure you want to get to the corner office, this book will help you decide. If you have already decided—this book will help you get there."

–*Lou Kacyn*
Partner, Egon Zehnder International

"As she did with our students, Fitzpatrick continues to impart wisdom, joining Curran to share their experiences and distill the advice of notable leaders to reveal the essence of leadership. This easy-to-read and inspirational book is a fundamental volume for all leadership courses and for those willing to take the risk and reap the reward of leadership."

–*Terri E. Weaver, PhD, RN, FAAN*
Dean, College of Nursing
Professor of Biobehavioral and Health Science
University of Illinois at Chicago

"Curran and Fitzpatrick, authors of *Claiming the Corner Office,* provide nurse leaders with encouragement to take bold actions. Their first-of-its-kind book includes real-world success strategies and pearls of wisdom from nurse executives who have claimed the corner office. These success stories motivate nurse leaders to stop doubting their own abilities, so they too can rightfully claim the corner office. I'd advise nurse leaders to use this book as a road map to the corner office."

–*Beth A. Brooks, PhD, RN, FACHE*
President, Resurrection University

"The authors recognize the personal qualities that make a great nurse and provide a road map that uses these qualities to obtain leadership success. Their lessons are specific, concrete, and adaptable. An absolute must-read for graduate nursing students and experienced nurses wishing to develop their career path in leadership, this book recognizes the importance of having the right person in the corner office and supplies the tools to get there."

–Janice Gries, DNP, RNC, IBCLC, APN
President, JCG Healthcare, LLC

"This book is first rate and long overdue. Curran and Fitzpatrick are, at their core, passionate teachers, and *Claiming the Corner Office* is a must-read for every nurse planning a career of consequence. They write to inspire and guide current and future leaders to achieve at extraordinary levels. Illustrated with compelling stories, the book describes the need to plan while leaving room for serendipity. This book is useful on both a personal and professional level."

–Sharon O'Keefe
President, University of Chicago Medical Center

Claiming the Corner Office

Executive Leadership Lessons for Nurses

Connie Curran, EdD, RN, FAAN
Therese Fitzpatrick, PhD, RN

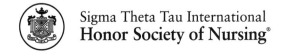

Sigma Theta Tau International
Honor Society of Nursing®

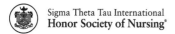

Sigma Theta Tau International
Honor Society of Nursing®

The Honor Society of Nursing, Sigma Theta Tau International (STTI) is a nonprofit organization whose mission is to support the learning, knowledge, and professional development of nurses committed to making a difference in health worldwide. Founded in 1922, STTI has more than 130,000 active members in more than 85 countries. Members include practicing nurses, instructors, researchers, policymakers, entrepreneurs, and others. STTI's 486 chapters are located at 662 institutions of higher education throughout Australia, Botswana, Brazil, Canada, Colombia, England, Ghana, Hong Kong, Japan, Kenya, Malawi, Mexico, the Netherlands, Pakistan, Singapore, South Africa, South Korea, Swaziland, Sweden, Taiwan, Tanzania, the United States, and Wales. More information about STTI can be found online at www.nursingsociety.org.

Sigma Theta Tau International
550 West North Street
Indianapolis, IN, USA 46202

To order additional books, buy in bulk, or order for corporate use, contact Nursing Knowledge International at 888.NKI.4YOU (888.654.4968/US and Canada) or +1.317.634.8171 (outside US and Canada).

To request a review copy for course adoption, email solutions@nursingknowledge.org or call 888. NKI.4YOU (888.654.4968/US and Canada) or +1.317.634.8171 (outside US and Canada).

To request author information, or for speaker or other media requests, contact Rachael McLaughlin of the Honor Society of Nursing, Sigma Theta Tau International at 888.634.7575 (US and Canada) or +1.317.634.8171 (outside US and Canada).

ISBN: 9781937554354
EPUB ISBN: 9781937554514
PDF ISBN: 9781937554521
MOBI ISBN: 9781937554538

Library of Congress Cataloging-in-Publication Data

Curran, Connie L.
  Claiming the corner office : executive leadership lessons for nurses / Connie Curran, Therese Fitzpatrick.
    p. ; cm.
  Includes bibliographical references.
  ISBN 978-1-937554-35-4 (print : alk. paper) -- ISBN 978-1-937554-51-4 (ePUB) -- ISBN 978-1-937554-52-1 (PDF) (print) -- ISBN 978-1-937554-53-8 (MOBI)
  I. Fitzpatrick, Therese, 1953- II. Sigma Theta Tau International. III. Title.
  [DNLM: 1. Nurse Administrators. 2. Leadership. 3. Nurse's Role. 4. Organizational Culture. 5. Staff Development. WY 105]
  RT49
  362.17'30684--dc23
                        2013002985

First Printing, 2013

Publisher: Renee Wilmeth
Acquisitions Editor: Emily Hatch
Editorial Coordinator: Paula Jeffers
Cover Designer: Michael Tanamachi
Interior Design/Page Layout: Katy Bodenmiller

Principal Book Editor: Carla Hall
Content Editor: John Curley
Project Editor: Kevin Kent
Proofreader: Erin Geile
Indexer: Jane Palmer

Dedication

This book is dedicated to my father, Patrick Curran, whose Wisconsin Wisdom included "If you are not the lead dog, the view is always the same," and "You either own or are owned." His inspiration motivated me to the corner office.

–Connie

For Alan, who persistently reminded me that passion was the primary requisite for a successful journey to the corner office.

–Therese

Finally, this book is dedicated to those nurses who dreamed big and took the bold steps required to gain access to the corner office. They are truly game changers.

It is also dedicated to those nurses with aspirations to become the next generation of nurse entrepreneurs, inventors, and corner office leaders as they dare to transform cultures and reinvent the old ways of doing business in health care.

Acknowledgments

We have been very fortunate to work with many talented colleagues while writing this book. The nurse leaders who shared their stories with us and the many mentors, employers, employees, and patients who've worked with us during the years were a constant source of inspiration.

We are especially grateful to Linda Pophal for her hard work, perseverance, and belief in our idea.

The leaders of Sigma Theta Tau have been enthusiastic supporters of the book. Carla Hall, Emily Hatch, and Kevin Kent were enormously helpful in creating this book.

Finally, we are grateful to our children for the joy and inspiration that they have provided throughout our careers.

About the Authors
Connie Curran, EdD, RN, FAAN

Connie Curran is the CEO of Best On Board, a national organization focused on educating and certifying health care trustees. She was the founding executive director of C-Change, a national organization focused on the eradication of cancer. C-Change participants, approximately 150 in all, included the heads of federal and state governmental agencies, for-profit corporations, the motion picture industry, and nonprofit groups whose missions relate to cancer. Former President George H. W. Bush and Barbara Bush served as cochairs, with Senator Dianne Feinstein serving as vice chair.

Curran was the founder, president, and chief executive officer of CurranCare, LLC, from 1995 to 2000. CurranCare was a national management and consulting services organization that delivered dynamic leadership to the health care industry. Cardinal Health acquired CurranCare, and Curran served as president of Cardinal Health Consulting Services, providing leadership to approximately 200 consultants.

Curran has held a variety of executive positions in academic and health care organizations: She was the chief nursing officer of Montefiore Medical Center in the Bronx; vice president of the American Hospital Association, where she was the first executive director of the American Organization of Nurse Executives; and dean at the Medical College of Wisconsin.

Curran is also one of the most prolific scholars in the field, with more than 200 publications and several research programs to her credit. She served as the director of two of the most comprehensive national studies on staff recruitment, retention, and labor market participation. More recently, she has co-authored books on hospital-physician integration, hospital redesign, and optimized home care integration. She served as the editor of *Nursing Economic$* for 18 years and now serves as the editor emeritus.

In addition to having held faculty and administrative positions at several universities, Curran is a faculty member of the American College of Healthcare Executives. She is a graduate of the Harvard Business School program for company owners and presidents. She serves on the board of directors for Hospira, Inc.; DeVry, Inc.; DePaul University; and Larkin Street and is a former chairman of the board of Silver Cross Hospital.

Therese Fitzpatrick, PhD, RN

Therese Fitzpatrick is the executive vice president of Assay Healthcare Solutions, a New York-based, investor-backed consulting and analytics firm focused on the use of mathematical optimization modeling in strategic clinical workforce planning and deployment. This innovative company, which has a nationwide client base, achieved profitability prior to projections. The company has been built around the science of logistics and the adaptation of sophisticated tools and techniques used with great success in a multitude of other industries outside of health care.

Fitzpatrick was also a founding partner of The Optimé Group, a self-funded company that provided technology solutions and business process support services that enabled health care clients to improve decision-making and optimize critical processes. She first ventured into the corner office as the CEO of a successful, private equity-owned nurse staffing company in Chicago. After growing its revenues to more than $8 million annually, she facilitated a merger with another staffing company to form the largest regional clinical staffing organization in Chicago, doubling revenues within the first year. Within this company, she built a consulting division focused on providing innovative strategies for hospitals related to demand planning, staffing optimization, and dynamic budgeting.

She is also an assistant clinical professor at the University of Illinois-Chicago College of Nursing, Department of Health System Sciences, where she teaches graduate administrative studies. Her research interests include workforce productivity, complexity management, and systems theory. In addition to her faculty role, she is the director of consulting for the college's Institute for Health Care Innovation. She has served in the role of chief nursing officer and chief operating officer in both academic and community health care systems, including a Top 100 hospital system.

Fitzpatrick recently presented the results of research on optimizing nursing human capital at the International Nursing Administration Research meeting, the Royal College of Surgeons in Ireland, and the annual meeting of the American Organization of Nurse Executives. Her work on human capital optimization was awarded the Greatest Potential Contribution to Nursing Practice by the Royal College. Her work on optimization modeling was published in February 2010 in the *Journal of Nursing Administration*. She and a colleague at UIC have recently published a chapter in the fourth edition of Huber's *Leadership and Nursing Care Management* focused on financial management and a 2009 article in the *Journal of Nursing Administration* describing research focused on the elimination of non value-added activities for staff nurses.

Fitzpatrick serves on several boards of directors, including the editorial board of the journal *Nursing Economic$*; chair of the Good Samaritan Hospital Governance Council, a Malcolm Baldrige recipient, in Downers Grove, Illinois; Turning Point Community Mental Health Center, Skokie, Illinois; and as an advisor to the metro-Chicago Women Health Executive Network. She received her PhD in urban studies at the University of Wisconsin-Milwaukee. Her research interest is in the creation of community through community planning and architecture. She received her BSN from DePaul University in Chicago along with her MS in nursing administration, with a particular focus in human resource management and labor relations.

Fitzpatrick is also a member of Amnesty International's specialty group for health care professionals and has participated in international community needs assessments.

About the Contributors

Rhonda Anderson, RN, DNSc(h), FAAN, FACHE

Rhonda Anderson is chief executive officer of Cardon Children's Medical Center in Mesa, Arizona. She is a fellow in the American Academy of Nursing and the American College of Healthcare Executives (ACHE). She served as the Joint Commission commissioner for 9 years. She was on the board of JCI and was the ACHE regent for Arizona. She also serves on the Institute for Interactive Patient Care National Advisory Board, National Guideline Clearinghouse and National Quality Measures Clearinghouse Expert Panel, American Hospital Association Board of Trustees, American Hospital Association Health Research and Educational Trust Board and Committee on Research, National Association of Children's Hospitals and Related Institutions Quality Council, National Quality Forum Measure Applications Partnership Coordinating Committee, and Robert Wood Johnson Foundation National Advisory Committee/Academic Progression in Nursing Program. She has been involved as a member or chair of state and national patient safety and quality committees and performance measurement committees over the past 10 years. Anderson is trustee of the Arizona Perinatal Trust and chairman of the board of directors for Children's Action Alliance.

Anderson received the Distinguished Achievement Award from Arizona State University, College of Nursing, and was a selected participant in the First International Institute: Executive Nurse Leadership in the United Kingdom and the United States, Florence Nightingale Trust in London, England. She attended the Wharton School of Business as a selected participant in the Johnson & Johnson Fellowship Program. In November 2005, Anderson was awarded the Nursing Legend, Nurse of the Year Award by the March of Dimes. Anderson was awarded the American Organization of Nurses Executives' Lifetime Achievement Award in April 2006 and *NurseWeek*'s Lifetime Achievement Award in September 2006, and she is a *Phoenix Business Journal* 2011 Women in Business honoree. Anderson was named *Arizona Business Magazine*'s 2012 Health Care Leadership Award

"Hospital Executive of the Year" and one of its "Fifty Most Influential Women in Arizona Business." She is also the recipient of the Association of Professional Chaplains 2012 Leadership Award "Distinguished Service Award." She is currently on four editorial boards of health care and nursing journals.

Ann Scott Blouin, PhD, RN, FACHE

Ann Scott Blouin is the executive vice president of customer relations at The Joint Commission. In this position, Blouin focuses on building and strengthening external customer and stakeholder relationships, primarily in the hospital market. She gathers customer input and feedback, assisting in guiding business development and retention strategies. In addition, she continues her leadership role with the Nursing Advisory Council and cosponsors the Health Systems Corporate Liaison group.

From 2008 to 2012, Blouin held the position of executive vice president for the Division of Accreditation and Certification Operations at The Joint Commission. Her responsibilities included executive leadership of accreditation and certification for more than 19,000 health care organizations and programs, including all activities related to surveys, eligibility and application processes, customer account management, and federal deeming compliance requirements. The Hospital, Critical Access Hospital, and Laboratory programs report through this division. Blouin also administered accreditation and certification policy development, surveyor education and development, survey technology, and the ongoing development and refinement of accreditation process components.

With more than 30 years of health care administration, consulting, and clinical nursing experience, Blouin has held positions of program administrator, vice president for nursing, and executive vice president for operations at two Chicago-area community teaching hospitals and a Chicago academic medical center. She has worked with multiple health systems across the United States to help them improve quality and patient safety, revenue management, and operating cost efficiency and effectiveness. Blouin has consulted with a large number of health care organizations, serving in leadership roles at consulting firms such as Ernst & Young LLP and Huron Consulting Group Inc. Prior to joining The Joint Commission in August 2008, Blouin was a principal at Deloitte, a national leader of management consulting services in patient safety, quality, and capacity management.

Blouin has published and taught extensively on topics focused on health care and nursing administration and has served as an adjunct faculty member at several Chicago-area schools of nursing and medicine. She currently serves on the National Patient Safety Foundation board of directors and as an editorial advisor for the *Journal of Nursing Administration* and *Biotechnology Healthcare.*

Blouin earned her PhD in nursing sciences and MBA from the University of Illinois at Chicago. She received her MSN with honors in maternal/child nursing from Loyola University of Chicago, and BSN with high honors from Lewis University in Romeoville, Illinois. She is a fellow of the American College of Healthcare Executives and member of the American Organization of Nurse Executives, American Nurses Association, and the Honor Society of Nursing, Sigma Theta Tau International.

Paula Lucey, MSN, RN

Paula Lucey is administrator of the Milwaukee County Behavioral Health Division. This division includes an acute care mental health hospital, nursing home, facility for the cognitively disabled, and an extensive network of crisis and community resources. She has expertise in developing systems of care for the uninsured in communities as well as in creating community partnerships.

Lucey has had an extensive career in health care and nursing leadership. She was the chief nursing officer and associate hospital administrator for patient care services at the John L. Doyne Hospital; creator and administrator of the General

Assistance Medical Program, which was a prototype managed care program for the uninsured; and director of health and human services for Milwaukee County.

She has been recognized for her leadership with the Quality Innovation Award from the American Organization of Nurse Executives and the Nursing Administrative Leadership award from *Nursing Economic$*.

Lucey is a graduate of the University of Wisconsin-Milwaukee College of Nursing, which recognized her with an alumni award. She received a master's degree in nursing administration from Marquette University, which also recognized her with an alumni award.

She received several fellowships, including the Johnson & Johnson Wharton Nurse Executive Fellowship and the Robert Wood Johnson Executive Nurse Fellowship.

Lucey also serves her community as a member of the local board of health and a member of the board of directors for a Federally Qualified Health Center.

Patricia O'Donoghue, PhD, PNP

Patricia O'Donoghue is interim provost of DePaul University. A scholar and teacher with broad clinical and research experience, she served as president of Mount Mary College in Milwaukee, Wisconsin, from 1997 to 2006. She was vice president for academic affairs and professor of nursing at La Roche College in Pittsburgh, Pennsylvania, from 1995 to 1997 and was provost and executive vice president at Carlow University in Pittsburgh from 1992 to 1997.

She was a member of the founding faculty of the School Nurse Practitioner Program at Carlow University and held clinical and faculty positions at Indiana University of Pennsylvania, University of Pittsburgh, Magee-Womens Hospital, and Children's Hospital of Pittsburgh.

O'Donoghue, who holds a doctorate in nursing from the University of Pittsburgh, has received numerous accolades for leadership, including the YWCA Wisconsin Women of Distinction Award; the School Sisters of Notre Dame-Milwaukee Province Special Achievement Award; and the Distinguished Alumni Award from the University of Pittsburgh School of Nursing.

She has served on the boards of many nonprofit schools and organizations, including the Foundation for Independent Higher Education, the Women's College Coalition, Foundation Rwanda, and the American Council on Education Commission on Women in Higher Education.

P. K. Scheerle, RN

P. K. Scheerle, RN, founded American Nursing Services (ANS), a privately held, highly successful nurse staffing company in 1982. Under her direction, the company grew from five employees to more than 2,500 employees with locations in nine states, providing local nurse staffing, travel nurses, therapists, and private duty nurses. During her tenure, ANS received numerous awards, including the American Business Ethics Award from the Society of Financial Service Professionals, a Top 100 Business by *New Orleans CityBusiness* for 11 consecutive years, and America's Top 500 Women-Owned Business by *Working Women Magazine*.

Scheerle, an RN with a clinical background in pediatric intensive care, is a self-made entrepreneur who saw a need in the nursing industry to keep experienced and talented nurses at the bedside. By utilizing her remarkable vision and tremendous determination, she created one of the nation's leading nurse supplemental staffing companies.

Scheerle graduated from the Executive Program of Harvard Business School in 1991 after graduating from nursing school in 1980 as president of her class.

Scheerle has served and continues to serve on numerous for-profit and not-for-profit boards. She has also received many awards for contributions to the community and the nursing profession including, but not limited to, the Humanitarian of the Year Award from the Southeast Chapter of the American Red Cross, induction into the Junior Achievement Business Hall of Fame, the Boggs-Bourque Woman of Distinction Award, and the *New Orleans CityBusiness* Women of the Year Award for 3 consecutive years. She also served as chairman of the Young Presidents' Organization for Louisiana and served on its Southern Regional Board.

In addition, Scheerle continues to be in great demand as a consultant and speaker for businesses, entrepreneurships, and value creation. She is regularly sought after and relied upon for her expertise by successful CEOs.

She is married to Bruce Bolyard, and they have three daughters and a son.

Roy Simpson, DNP, RN, DPNAP, FAAN

Roy Simpson, vice president of nursing informatics at Cerner Corporation, is responsible for executive leadership in nursing and relationships for the global patient care enterprise as well as representation at the industry level for Cerner's nurse practice.

Simpson has more than 30 years of experience in nursing informatics and in senior executive administration. His primary executive research focus pioneered the development and funding of the Werley and Lang Nursing Minimum Data Set (NMDS). The NMDS is a minimum set of nursing data elements with uniform definitions and categories, including nursing problems, diagnoses, interventions, and patient outcomes, approved by the American Nurses Association. Simpson joined Cerner Corporation in 2000.

He has served on the board of trustees for Excelsior College, formerly Regents College, at the State University of New York, where he established the Roy L. Simpson Nursing Informatics Scholarship. In 2001, he served as the Frances and Earl Ziegler Visiting Scholar at the University of Oklahoma and as the Merle Lott Distinguished Lecturer at Georgia State University. He served as distinguished professor at the University of Wales during the European Summer School on Nursing Informatics in 2002. He received the Informatics Award from Rutgers University in 1999 and the Maes MacInnis Award from New York University in 2003. In 2007, Simpson was awarded honorary international membership in the International Medical Informatics Association and also honorary membership in the Honor Society of Nursing, Sigma Theta Tau International, representing his scholarship and his contribution to the field of informatics.

Simpson lectures extensively around the world and has published more than 500 articles on nursing informatics and executive leadership. He also sits on 12 editorial review boards. He is a fellow of the American Academy of Nursing, where he served as chair of the expert panel on Nursing Informatics and Technology. He is an active member of numerous professional organizations—ANA, AMIA, NLN, AONE, NI-WIG, and CARING. In addition, he holds status as a fellow in the New York Academy of Medicine and a distinguished practitioner in the National Academies of Practice. He attained a doctorate in nursing practice, executive leadership/informatics, at American Sentinel University.

Patricia E. Thompson, EdD, RN, FAAN

Patricia E. Thompson is the chief executive officer for the Honor Society of Nursing, Sigma Theta Tau International (STTI). In this position, she leads the staff in implementing the board's vision for this 130,000-member organization during a time of unprecedented global expansion. She develops and strengthens relationships with internal and external stakeholders worldwide.

She has also served in many volunteer leadership roles for STTI, including president (1999-2001) and chair of the board of directors of both the International Honor Society of Nursing Building Corporation and Nursing Knowledge International, STTI subsidiaries.

Thompson has been involved in many international programs and initiatives, including Sigma Theta Tau International's Arista3 conferences. These multinational, multidisciplinary conferences served as "think tanks." The focus was to create nursing's preferred future for healthy communities globally.

Thompson has more than 35 years of experience in health care and academic consulting, teaching, and administration. She served as a consultant for Sunbeam-Oster Housewares at its Louisiana plant. Maternity and nursery costs were decreased by 86%. Details about the program were reported nationally, including *The Wall Street Journal*, *Businessweek*, and *Good Morning America*.

Thompson has been an investigator for more than 20 grant-funded programs, including a workforce diversity grant from the Health Resources and Services Administration to support minorities in nursing. She has numerous publications and presentations on leadership, scholarship, maternal-child issues, and nursing education. She has also served on professional and community boards. She has received many honors and awards, including the Athena Award, recognizing excellence in business, service, and leadership, from the Chamber of Commerce.

In the early 1970s, Thompson obtained her BSN from Northwestern State University (Natchitoches, Louisiana) and an MSN in pediatrics from the University of Alabama in Birmingham. In the early 1980s, she returned to the classroom and earned her EdD in higher education administration with a minor in business management from the University of North Texas (Denton, Texas). Her clinical career began in pediatric staff nursing prior to moving into academics.

Table of Contents

Introduction

> *"Leadership is not magnetic personality; that can just as well be a glib tongue. It is not 'making friends and influencing people'; that is flattery. Leadership is lifting a person's vision to higher sights, the raising of a person's performance to a higher standard, the building of a personality beyond its normal limitations."*
>
> *–Peter Drucker*

There is a quiet revolution underway. The initials "RN" are appearing on nameplates on corner office doors, and the impact of nurses' intellectual capital is becoming evident in strategic decision-making in boardrooms, the public policy arena, and businesses across the nation. Smart, bold, and exceedingly qualified nurses are blazing trails into domains once reserved for the daring entrepreneur, venture capitalist, or pin-striped business school graduate. The time has come to celebrate and study these nursing successes. Their accomplishments deserve to be hailed, because these unique leaders have done what was considered highly unlikely even 30 years ago. These leaders have embraced their valuable nursing knowledge and their unique perspective on health and health care and leveraged this expertise in pursuit of the most strategic and powerful positions in universities, government, health care organizations, and corporate enterprises.

Their stories must be told, because they are breaking through barriers once thought of as impenetrable for nurses. But more importantly, we need to understand how they did it so that we can begin to shape the science around this level of sophisticated leadership, building our capacity as nurses and positioning others for inclusion in these unique ranks. Capturing the important lessons from their storied careers will form the basis for curricula in our executive graduate programs and provide the models for others as they contemplate their own corner office journeys.

Perhaps the most meaningful aim in conveying these valuable experiences is the hope that it will assure you, the reader, that these opportunities are available to you—that like these corner office executives, you, too, possess the capacity to develop your careers in extraordinary directions. These remarkable role models have taught us that the skills and competencies required to journey into the corner office can be learned and practiced, so that you become confident and secure in your abilities and able to compete for these coveted positions.

You are poised at a unique time to make meaningful contributions not only to your organization but also to the health care industry as a whole. Health care costs have an enormous impact on this country, as you well know. Health care costs consume 18% of our gross domestic product and are the largest single budget item in every state. The federal government, state governments, employers, employees, insurers, and citizens are all demanding lower health care costs—with higher quality care.

Our industry is in the midst of chaos as we attempt to manage the uncertainty of reform, disquiet in Congress, shrinking reimbursement, and perhaps the largest change to the model of care ever experienced in health care, as the epicenter of care shifts into the community. Yet, history has demonstrated that from chaos, opportunity is born. Creative nurse entrepreneurs, intrapreneurs, and innovative leaders have embraced this complexity and are beginning to reinvent their organizations and themselves to meet the challenge.

As the largest group of health care professionals, nurses possess the greatest breadth and depth of health care experience in hospitals, clinics, long-term care, and the home. Nurses are a tremendous source of information on how to lower costs and improve quality. They are an enormous asset to entrepreneurs and corporations in creating products and processes that will lead to lower costs and higher quality care. The experience of nursing, the passionate mission for patients and caregivers, creativity, and persistence combine to create great executives who are successful in the corner office.

Unfortunately, we will not be revealing any magic formulae to speed the journey, for everyone's journey will be different. And much of your eventual success will be dependent on your personal failures and disappointments, as well as on your ability to turn those defeats into subsequent successes. Like our favorite football team (that would be the Green Bay Packers for Connie), your success will depend on how skilled you are at watching the game tapes, evaluating the plays where yardage was lost, and applying those learnings toward a successful drive to the goal the following week. As you are about to learn, it's all about learning from our missteps and becoming stronger leaders as a result.

You are also about to learn that the route to the corner office is circuitous, with interesting detours and side trips. You might face stops along the route to raise families, perform voluntary service, or even to join a spouse in an overseas assignment. Nonetheless, these experiences also become part of the repertoire of proficiencies and life lessons that propel us along our journey.

Roy Simpson, vice president for nursing informatics at Cerner Corporation, reminded us that the corner office in this era of global industrialization and telecommuting might not actually be located in the corner of the C-suite (a widely used slang term used to collectively refer to a corporation's most important senior executives) at all. You will find executive nurses managing employees across the nation, managing contracts with vendors across the globe, and leading campuses in nations thousands of miles from their corner office. They are conducting strategy sessions virtually with translators as standing members of their team and managing multimillion dollar enterprises from their home offices. And though the 21st-century office might look uniquely different from the traditional corporate suite, the characteristics and competencies of the executives ensconced in those offices have radically changed as well. These times that offer so much opportunity for the innovative executive require a 21st-century skill set, as business as usual will no longer be tolerated.

The authors have spent an inordinate amount of time on airplanes, or waiting for airplanes, while traversing the country for business. The average flight time for a cross-country trip has become a metric by which we measure time and our productivity. We have come to know how many pages of a consulting report can be written on a Chicago to New York City flight or precisely how many journals to grab off the desk for a Denver to San Francisco flight. As a result, we wanted to write a book that could be consumed on a Boston to Las Vegas flight. This is not a textbook, quite intentionally. We hope that you will have fun reading this book, because we truly enjoyed writing it and found tremendous inspiration from talking with the remarkable nurses whose experiences you will find within these pages.

The leaders described on these pages could not be more different. Some are thoughtful and measure each word precisely, some are scholarly, and still others are spontaneous; yet, the similarities in their career trajectories and professional outlooks are startlingly similar. Though they might be occupying corner offices in very different types of organizations, the experiential priorities and requisite skills they identified as necessary for their journeys were universal.

We will pepper the pages with their stories, advice, and candid accounts of both successes and failures. We will also attempt to convey their personal challenges in managing two-career families and how their voices wavered when describing a missed soccer game or having to miss an important board meeting, because they just *couldn't* miss another soccer game. Yet, it was precisely because of these experiences and the need to juggle a lifetime of multiple priorities that they became the resilient, understanding, and unstoppable leaders that they are.

The contemporary enterprise is decidedly more chaotic as information for decision-making becomes more abundant, consumers of all services and products become more demanding, regulations become more stringent, and feedback becomes more public, thanks to the Internet. In this book, we will also attempt to provide relevant management theory and background information for those hoping to lead in these tumultuous times in what we hope will be a quick guide for your corner office journey map. Please indulge our informal (and often quite forthright and pragmatic) and individual writing styles.

It is our sincere hope that you will find inspiration in the careers of the corner office executives interviewed for this work and that you can visualize your name on that plate on the door of the corner office.

> *"Making your mark in the world is hard. If it were easy everybody would do it. But it's not. It takes patience, it takes commitment and it comes with plenty of failure along the way. The real test is not whether you avoid failure, because you won't. It's whether you let it harden or shame you into inaction, or whether you learn from it; whether you choose to persevere."*
>
> *–Barack Obama*

Chapter 1

The New Frontier: Nurses in the Executive Suite

"If you feel that you've failed in something, just sit back and in 2, 3, or 4 years, after some time has passed and you can reflect on it, there are some things you can learn. Take some level of comfort that even if you didn't get the chief nursing officer job or the chief executive officer job, or even if you get fired—which many of us have been fired—you learn to move on. You still learn something from those experiences."

–Ann Scott Blouin, September 2012

As a child in a military family, Pat Thompson quickly became used to change and adapting to new places and new situations. These early experiences shaped her approach to her career as she adapted to opportunities that came her way, ultimately building a career in education and administration that led her to the corner office at Sigma Theta Tau International (STTI), where she serves as CEO.

Education and administration were not originally part of her plans. When she graduated from high school she went straight into a nursing program; while nobody from her family was a nurse, she had a passion to "help people," she says. But, during her junior year a faculty mentor asked her if she had ever thought about teaching as a profession. "My answer was 'absolutely not!'" she says. "But, I thought about it over time and decided I really did have an interest." Her mentor advised that she pursue her master's degree immediately after college, rather than working as a staff nurse, which was far more common at the time. She applied to and was accepted by the University of Alabama in Birmingham, because she was interested in pursuing a pediatrics track.

She became involved in the student nurses' association and was elected president of her chapter and, while attending her first state convention, was elected president of the state association when another candidate became ineligible. Her peers encouraged her to run against the other candidate, and although she felt unprepared for such a role, she did—and she was elected. Those early experiences positioned her well for the opportunity of becoming CEO of STTI. In the intervening years, she earned her doctorate, taught, and ultimately became interested in administration.

It was a disappointment that ultimately led her to the office she holds now. She had been at the University of Arkansas for Medical Sciences for about 16 years when the dean retired and the position became available. A national search was conducted, and she was one of two internal candidates for the position; the other candidate was awarded the job. It was a blow, but she committed not only to continuing in her role but to supporting the new dean. During this time, the CEO position at STTI opened.

"I never thought of ever being in this position," she says. "I never thought the position would open, for one thing." She did not apply. But, the search firm contacted her based on a recommendation that she would be a good candidate. "They called me and I still wasn't really sure," she says. There were two things that were a concern for her. One, "whether I could do the job or not, because I'd never done anything quite of this scope before." And, the second, the climate. "I had never intended to live anyplace that had snow on the ground for more than a day at a time," she laughs. But, after participating in a rigorous interview process that involved several rounds and several interviews, she was offered the job. "I eventually decided that this job was worth it, and I could learn the 'snow skill set,' which I have."

Importantly, she notes, "If I had gotten the dean job, I never would have considered this, because I wouldn't have left that position." Thompson's path to the corner office is not unlike that of other nurses who have attained roles in hospital, education, and entrepreneurial settings.

The world of nursing has changed considerably from the days when Florence Nightingale cared for wounded soldiers. Today, nurses can be found in settings ranging from the traditional hospital, to the classroom, to the boardroom, and multiple variations in between.

In addition to Pat Thompson, EdD, RN, FAAN, the nurses we interviewed while writing this book are:

- Rhonda Anderson, RN, DNSc(h), FAAN, FACHE, CEO at Cardon Children's Medical Center

- Paula Lucey, MSN, RN, administrator, Milwaukee County Behavioral Health

- Pat O'Donoghue, PhD, PNP, interim provost at DePaul University

- P. K. Scheerle, RN, CEO and chairman of Gifted Nurses

- Ann Scott Blouin, PhD, RN, FACHE, executive vice president of customer relations with The Joint Commission

- Roy Simpson, DNP, RN, DPNAP, FAAN, vice president of nursing informatics, Cerner Corporation

We share their insights with you throughout this book, as well as our own, drawn from our experiences and our current roles—Connie as CEO of Best on Board, a training and certification program for health care board members, and founder and former CEO of CurranCare, and Therese as executive vice president of Assay Healthcare Solutions. We know from our own career paths and those of the many other successful nurses we have encountered along the way that opportunities abound. Over the years, we have learned from our successes; importantly, we have often learned even more from our failures.

We believe that—with health care reform still looming, but uncertain in terms of its impact, and the nation's aging population destined to place an increasing burden on an already overburdened system—there has never been a better time for nurses to move into myriad leadership roles.

There could be a wealth of opportunities for nurses to move into positions of leadership as health care executives, policy-makers, government officials, and business leaders. Beverly Malone, PhD, RN, FAAN, head of the National League for Nursing, said, "This is your time!" (Robert Wood Johnson Foundation, 2011, p.1). According to the blog, among the factors driving new opportunity were last year's passage of a law overhauling the nation's health care system; the release of a groundbreaking Institute of Medicine (IOM) report calling on nurses to contribute as essential partners in the redesign of the nation's health care system (IOM, 2010); and the multifaceted Future of Nursing: Campaign for Action supported by the Robert Wood Johnson Foundation to implement the IOM report's recommendations.

In the Robert Wood Johnson Foundation blog (2011), Pamela Thompson, MS, RN, CENP, FAAN, CEO of the American Organization of Nurse Executives (AONE), says nurses have moved in recent decades beyond their traditional executive-level roles as chief nursing officers at health care organizations and are now more likely to hold broader and more senior executive-level positions inside and outside of health care organizations and systems.

The sheer variety of opportunities in nursing today makes the profession one that can hold infinite possibility for nurses, regardless of their areas of interest. Starting points are for nurses interested in corner office roles are understanding what is required in leadership roles and conducting a self-assessment to determine if they have the requisite skills.

Many Routes, One Set of Skills: What Does It Take?

In 1949, Estella Mann, RN, wrote "The Head Nurse as a Leader" (Mann, 1949). In it, she says, "Leadership implies the ability to direct and guide the actions of others" (p. 627) and points to "five important goals for the supervisor who wishes to improve her ability as a leader" (p. 627):

- Develop your employees' confidence in you.

- Develop your employees' confidence in themselves.

- Stimulate your employees' interest in their jobs.

- Treat your employees as individuals.

- Strive to improve your own ability as a supervisor.

It seems in 1949, the role of a leader was more like the role of a manager today. Here is a more recent and, we think, better definition of what leaders do. In 1989, Max DePree, CEO of Herman Miller, Inc., said that the first responsibility of a leader is to define reality (DePree, 1989). Even beyond that, successful leaders need to be able to *communicate* that reality to various constituents. AONE has outlined five leadership domains and related competencies, which are detailed in Table 1.1.

TABLE 1.1 Five Leadership Domains and Related Competencies

Communication and relationship-building competencies	Effective communication
	Relationship management
	Influence of behaviors
	Ability to work with diversity
	Shared decision-making
	Community involvement
	Medical staff relationships
	Academic relationship
Knowledge of the health care environment	Clinical practice knowledge
	Patient care delivery models and work design knowledge
	Health care economics knowledge
	Understanding of governance
	Understanding of evidence-based practice
	Outcome measurement
	Knowledge of and dedication to patient safety
	Understanding of utilization/case management
	Knowledge of risk management
Leadership skills	Foundational thinking skills
	Personal journey disciplines
	The ability to use systems thinking
	Succession planning
	Change management
Professionalism	Personal and professional accountability
	Career planning
	Ethics
	Evidence-based clinical and management practice
	Advocacy for the clinical enterprise and for nursing practice
	Active membership in professional organizations

Business skills	Understanding of health care financing
	Human resource management and development
	Strategic management
	Marketing
	Information management and technology

Information for the table derived from the American Association of Nurse Executives (2005).

Leaders must be adept at thinking conceptually, suggested Robert L. Katz in a now classic *Harvard Business Review* article, "Skills of an Effective Administrator" (*Harvard Business Review*, 1998). In it, he says, "Conceptual skill involves the ability to see the enterprise as a whole; it includes recognizing how the various functions of the organization depend on one another and how changes in any one part affect all the others; and it extends to visualizing the relationship of the individual business to the industry, the community, and the political, social, and economic forces of the nation as a whole" (p. 3).

Not to minimize the importance of effectively leading others, but what Katz describes is clearly a much bigger—and more impactful—role than focusing only on employees.

The Gallup organization has done a great deal of research on the issue of leadership. Gallup scientists have studied more than 1 million work teams and have conducted more than 50,000 in-depth interviews with leaders and more than 20,000 interviews with followers. In the book *Strength-Based Leadership*, authors Tom Rath and Barry Conchie use Gallup's discoveries to point to three traits of effective leaders (Rath & Conchie, 2009):

- They invest in strengths. This, perhaps counterintuitive, finding is an important one with implications for leaders as well as individuals. Many of us tend to focus on improving our weaknesses. Yet, Gallup research suggests that a focus on strengths is the way to go. In fact, they suggest, when managers focus on employees' strengths, the odds of employees becoming more engaged in their work and with the organization increase by eight times.

- They surround themselves with the right people and maximize the impact of the collective team. Top-performing teams have strengths in the areas of execution, influence, relationship-building, and strategic thinking.

- They understand their followers' needs. Those needs tend to be, according to Gallup: trust, compassion, stability, and hope.

For nurses, leadership roles may exist in a variety of areas—they may take on leadership roles that are clinical, administrative, educational, political, and entrepreneurial. While there are specific traits that allow nurses to excel in each of these areas, as we reflected on our own experiences and spoke with other nurses in leadership roles, we began to see some consistencies in terms of what it takes to achieve corner office-level success.

Networking and Building Relationships

"How you relate to people is key," says Pat Thompson. "I don't care what position you're in. Some people do it better than others; some do it more easily than others; some people don't do it well at all. You've really got to get some coaching and figure out how to hone in on that, because there's so much interface you do with stakeholders internally and externally that that is pretty much an essential."

Ann Scott Blouin notes that networking can also help to provide background in areas nurse leaders may not be well prepared to deal with through their formal education—such as finance. "One thing that I did early on, while at Northwestern, was to get to know the finance guys," she says. "I asked several of them to sit down with me with the income statement and the balance sheet and explain them to me." Those relationships served her well, she recalls. "I'm absolutely positive that I got the support I got when I went from nursing to administration because I had done that. The finance guys felt OK with me. I'm not sure I would have had that reception from my colleagues had I not taken some initiative to learn more about finance."

Pat Thompson set about purposefully to develop contacts and build a network that could help her achieve her goal of becoming a leader within STTI. "I decided that I would like to be president of the local chapter in Louisiana, so I ran and I didn't get it." She did not let that initial failure hold her back, though, and the next time around she was successful. Then she decided she would like to be president of the organization. To achieve that goal, she says, "I started to network with a lot of the leaders at Sigma Theta Tau. I tried to find people that were involved, and they were all very gracious and shared what they thought would be helpful." Those early experiences with STTI clearly positioned her well for the role she holds today.

"Networking is absolutely key," agrees Rhonda Anderson. "Some of that is within your own profession; some of that is within the community." One very valuable networking experience she had occurred while she was working on the East Coast, an environment that was very different from her Midwestern roots. "There were a group of men who were Harvard grads who had started what they called 'The Club,'" she recalls. "They did reviews of books and poetry on a monthly basis. They invited me to be in The Club! I was the only woman and certainly wasn't a Harvard or Yale graduate. But what fun we had, and how interesting it was!"

Self-Awareness

"I think being able to realistically and objectively assess your strengths and whether you call them weaknesses or areas of opportunity for improvement, I don't care," says Pat Thompson. "You have to know what it is you do well, so you can leverage that and what areas you need to develop further. When you identify those, you really need to then—either through mentors, through formal education, through continuing education, through whatever—you need to develop those skill sets."

Self-awareness also involves developing a comfort level for who you are. Rhonda Anderson stresses that nurses should be genuine: "Every person has some wonderful innate traits and learned traits and characteristics," she says. "Trying to be somebody else doesn't help. Be who you are, build on those strengths, and know the areas where you need growth."

Pat O'Donoghue echoes this thought. "One area that is important when dealing with others is that you act with integrity. It is critical that those with whom you work learn to trust you and your judgment. This is about honesty." Having a strong sense of self-awareness can help to develop that consistency between words and deeds and to establish honest, trusting relationships with those around you.

Being Open to New Opportunities

None of the nurse leaders we spoke to created a tangible plan for their career and stuck steadfastly to that plan. Instead, they all found that their greatest successes came through being open to the exciting new opportunities and options that invariably presented themselves.

Connie's success, she says, has been based to a large degree on being open to new experiences, new approaches, and new pathways. "I always felt like I was tight about my mission—that I wanted to make things better for patients and caregivers—but I was loose about how I was going to get there," she says. "I didn't ever feel like there was only one right way.

"You need to be invested in several things, which allows you some risk-taking. If you're broad in your interests and the way you invest your time and talent, you can take risks so that when something doesn't work out just right that's OK, because probably something in another part of your life will."

"I actually had wanted to be a teacher," recalls Ann Scott Blouin. "That was my first goal in life; I really was not interested in health care." But, when she was a young woman working in a retail environment, a friend of hers who was in nursing school wrote to her about her experiences in clinical practice taking care of a patient. "She talked about what it felt like to take care of a patient and help relieve his pain and make him feel better. It was literally like a lightening bolt. I thought maybe, rather than teaching, which was a very overcrowded field in the 1970s, maybe I ought to think about nursing as another helping profession."

Later, while working in a clinical role in pediatrics, she got a call about an opportunity to work in a nurse manager role. Still working on her master's and not entirely certain she could handle the financial aspects of the role, she was hesitant. But, she rose to the challenge. And, she recalls, "I got to do all kinds of growing. I started as a nurse manager of a large unit and got promoted to a director of nursing. I was in that role for about 5 or 6 years and I loved it."

Pat O'Donoghue had a similar experience. While in her fifth year of an entry-level management position, she was approached by physician colleagues who asked her to consider developing the pediatric nurse practitioner role in collaboration with the University of Pittsburgh School of Medicine. "I was both honored and intimidated by the responsibility," she says. But, she took it on and says, "As a result, I became one of the very earliest pediatric nurse practitioners in the state of Pennsylvania."

Paula Lucey says, "I sort of have this quaint philosophy about adventure. I personally think people spend way too much time worrying about the right thing to do when you need to take the alternative that's in front of you and make it golden, and be golden in that opportunity and help people see you as a person that takes things that aren't that great and make them golden."

Our nurses have also found that even failures or lost opportunities can lead to unexpected successes. That was Pat Thompson's experience and what led her to her current role as CEO of STTI.

Therese was part of a layoff situation early in her career and says, "I think that at some point, while it is an oftentimes painful and kind of unpleasant situation, being terminated from a job is a very important experience. It teaches you resilience. Being terminated does not need to be a devastating thing in nursing. There are so many opportunities for us."

The bottom line: Each and every experience along your career pathway may lead to new and rewarding opportunities. Being alert enough to see those opportunities and flexible enough to seize them has served many nurse leaders very well.

Financial Savvy

Financial savvy is critical for nurses in any role. We are in the business of caring, but it *is* a business. This country is truly looking at nursing to help us understand the value in health care and how to provide the highest value possible in a cost-effective way.

Connie learned the importance of finance early on in her career. "In one of my first early jobs, I had a nun who was my boss, the dean, and she gave me the talking to about 'no money, no mission.' She basically said, 'We've got to run the school of nursing in a way that allows us to bring in more money than we spend; we have to get good faculty who will help us keep the students and prepare great nurses.'" Nursing education programs are often inadequate in preparing nurses to understand that cost and quality are interdependent, and both are key nursing responsibilities.

Ann Scott Blouin says, "At McNeal I really learned how to manage budgets and manage product lines, and that was not something I learned at Northwestern. At McNeal you had to learn to operate and do business decisions based on sound business logic, return on investment, return on assets, and that was very good learning for me."

Roy Simpson, based on his unique experience in the for-profit sector, notes that it is very important for nurses to move beyond an understanding of profit and loss—to an understanding of revenue production. "Nurse executives who are chief nursing executives (CNEs) of any of the systems, unless they've had revenue production experience, cannot move over into the medical industrial complex for an executive job. It's what kills them. They want to do budget control. But, the corporation, especially in sales, works in revenue. All of our stock quotes are based on how much revenue we can pull in. You earn your credibility by bringing in your revenue."

Navigating the Political Landmines

Politics exist at every level in every organization around the world. Nurses, whether in hospitals, universities, or private industry, must become adept at moving ideas and initiatives forward, sometimes when faced with what seem to be overwhelming obstacles.

Therese excels at this. Much of her career has been spent in organized hospitals, doing turnarounds with difficult labor relations situations. "As a result," she says, "I've learned mutual gains bargaining and win-win bargaining." She teaches these skills now and was certified in labor relations through Harvard's program.

"Mutual gains bargaining is really about 'how do both of us win, and how do we figure out how to work together for a bigger organizational goal?'" she says. "Those skills, while they're incredibly important in the HR/labor side of the world, have served me well in every single aspect of my career."

Roy Simpson's experience in the for-profit world has given him a perspective that many do not have. "I truly believe that, in corporate America, they can fire you any day you walk in the door. So I'm always ready for it. Being naïve is no longer accepted. In this complex business world, you can't be naïve."

With a career that has been spent entirely in the public sector, Paula Lucey notes that politics was a given and that developing solid political skills with both a "big P and a little p" was essential for her career. She recalls conversations with a director of labor relations she worked with. "He used to say, 'If you don't think you work in a political setting, just look at the name on the top of your paycheck. You work for a government. You work in a political setting. You've got to learn about politics.'" Her ability to navigate both the big and little realms of politics served her well, she said, as did the many relationships she established over the course of her career.

"I was lucky enough to negotiate our nursing contract a couple of times," says Lucey. "That really gave me a sense of it's not the nurses' contract, it's our contract. We got things; we gave up things. That was very helpful to me in terms of managing the nurses and thinking through organizationally how you'd managed your workforce a little bit. I think it's ultimately about relationships."

Never Giving Up

Finally, successful nurses have been successful at facing adversity—in many cases viewing adversity as a challenge that can be effectively overcome, even leveraged.

As Connie notes, "My mother used to say, 'there's more than one way to skin a cat,' so I learned to be creative. I learned there were lots of solutions to problems and you just had to talk to people, and read, and figure it out."

But, despite expanding opportunities, nurses, unfortunately, must often face old and outdated biases and perceptions about the roles they are prepared to take on in a leadership capacity. In 2009, Gallup interviewed 1,504 opinion leaders across key roles and industries. Their findings are distressing but point to opportunities for nurses. According to the Robert Wood Johnson Foundation, "The new survey finds that opinion leaders . . . view nurses as one of the most trusted sources of health information, but see nurses as having less influence on health care reform than government, insurance and pharmaceutical executives and others" (Robert Wood Johnson Foundation, 2010, para. 2). Yet, the piece goes on to say, "A strong majority of respondents say nurses should have more influence than they do now on health policy, planning and management" (para. 2).

Other key findings from the new Gallup survey:

- Opinion leaders feel that nurses' primary areas of influence are reducing medical errors (51%), improving quality of care (50%), and coordinating patient care in the health care system (40%).

- Large majorities of opinion leaders said they would like to see nurses have more influence in a large number of areas, including reducing medical errors and improving patient safety (90%); improving quality of care (89%); promoting wellness and expanding preventive care (86%); improving health care efficiency and reducing costs (84%); coordinating care through the health care system (83%); helping the health care system adapt to an aging population (83%); and increasing access to health care (74%).

- Seventy-five percent of opinion leaders said government officials will have a great deal of influence in health reform in the next 5 to 10 years, compared with 56% for insurance executives, 46% for pharmaceutical executives, 46% for health care executives, 37% for doctors, 20% for patients, and 14% for nurses.

- Opinion leaders identified the top barriers to nurses' increased influence and leadership as not being perceived as important decision-makers (69%) or revenue generators (68%) compared with doctors; nurses' focus on primary rather than preventive care (62%); and nursing not having a single voice in speaking on national issues (56%).

These are misconceptions that nurses must address as they seek to fill leadership roles in various settings. Throughout this book, we will be discussing ways to overcome these barriers through specific actions that can help nurses gain credibility as business leaders that can have an impactful role on their decision-making and revenue-impacting abilities.

The successful nurses we interviewed all shared one very interesting trait—they were all opportunistic when it came to taking advantage of the experiences that came their way. While some started with a general direction in mind, all agreed that success is often driven by unexpected opportunities that pop up along the way.

Unique Characteristics of Female Leaders

There are almost 3 million licensed registered nurses in the United States; of these, approximately 170,000 are men, representing only about 6% of the overall nursing population (Health Resources and Services Administration, 2004). While we will be focusing on leadership opportunities for both male and female nurses in this book, given the preponderance of women in these roles, it is important to point out some distinct differences between male and female leadership styles.

In 1990, Sally Helgesen wrote *The Female Advantage*, based on her study of the differences in how males and females lead organizations. In conducting her research, Helgesen (1995) observed meetings, listened to phone calls and conferences, and read correspondence. Based on these "diary studies," she documented how female leaders make decisions, schedule their days, gather and share information, motivate others, delegate, structure their companies, and hire and fire staff.

The "big difference" between men and women in leadership roles? Women tend to focus more on relationships. A female CEO who receives a letter from someone saying, "I'm looking for a job" will likely respond to the letter with a bit of advice and a few helpful suggestions. A male CEO would be more likely to throw the letter in the trash if not looking for someone to hire. Her studies revealed that in terms of time spent, women spent about the same amount of time managing outside relationships as men and about the same amount of time with their boards as men. The difference was women's focus on relationships. That, suggests Helgesen, can be an advantage for women. More often, though, women are impacted by subtle disadvantages that can be detrimental to their career trajectories.

Kathryn McDonagh, FACHE, and Nancy Paris, FACHE, recently wrote an article in which they talk about the various barriers faced by women, which ultimately serve to create large disparities over time in terms of salary, promotion, and prestige when compared with their male colleagues (McDonagh & Paris, 2012). They suggest that women's path to leadership is far more complex and "circuitous" than men's, resulting in a "leadership labyrinth." They point out, though, that this should not be viewed as a negative, but as a unique opportunity to build wisdom as they navigate each ring of the labyrinth, gaining knowledge and experience that can be particularly suited to transformational leadership roles. The Leadership Labyrinth Model (see Table 1.2) consists of seven concentric rings of personal development and related areas of personal inquiry and professional focus.

TABLE 1.2 The Leadership Labyrinth Model

RING	PERSONAL INQUIRY	PROFESSIONAL FOCUS
Competence	How do I prepare myself for a career in health care?	Education, skill, experience
Connectivity	How do I interface with others to learn, grow, and develop?	Networks, mentors, sponsors, advisors
Service	What contributions can I make that enhance my profession and community?	Volunteering, mentoring, teaching, publishing
Awareness	What am I doing that may impede my progress and fulfillment?	360-degree feedback, ethics, honest appraisal, moments of truth
Creation	Am I approaching my career in a way that brings out the best in me and others?	Integrity, collective impact, service above self, clarity of purpose
Renewal	How do I cultivate and sustain my passion and purpose?	Coaching, hobbies, family time, worship, solitude
Wisdom	How do I draw on my knowledge, awareness and experience to promote health and foster transformation?	Conscious choices, intentionality, service to humanity

Reprinted from McDonagh and Paris, 2012.

The terrain is different for women in health care, and that can both benefit and detract from their ability to position themselves for senior leadership roles. The detractions come from the misperceptions that still exist about nurses and the roles more appropriate for them. The benefits, though, come from continuing research to suggest that women are uniquely positioned to take on leadership roles because of their relationship-focused transformational leadership styles. That does not mean that our male colleagues are left with a disadvantage. Both male and female nurses must learn to move outside their comfort zones if their current actions and behaviors are barriers to moving on to bigger and better things.

Getting Outside of Your Comfort Zone

Neither we nor any of the nurses we interviewed for this book ever knew with 100% certainty that we would succeed in any of the roles we took on throughout our careers. In fact, if any of us had stayed in roles in which we were comfortable, none of us would be where we are now.

One of the key differentiators between those who become contenders for the corner office and those who remain in staff roles is the willingness to take risks, to try new things, and to sometimes take on roles and projects that really are beyond their comfort zones.

Suppose you are faced with a decision or a choice between two or more options. How do you determine what to do? One recommendation we have heard is to consider the "worst-case scenario." What is the worst thing that could happen if you do this thing? Push yourself to think of the worst, the worst, the worst! In most situations, for most people, the worst that could happen is you might make a fool out of yourself. You might fail. You might waste your time, or your money, or both.

But the scenario is often different for nurses. For nurses, the worst-case scenario is often that we might hurt or kill a patient. What could be worse than that? As nurses, this tends to be our mind-set, and it is certainly understandable. But think about it. When you are not dealing with patient issues, but with management or leadership issues, you are not going to hurt or kill anyone. You might make a fool of yourself. You might fail. But weigh those options against killing a patient, and suddenly you may see that the risk is really not that risky after all.

If you have never made a fool of yourself, now is the time. Get over it—do it! In a 1990 editorial in *Science*, Harold T. Shapiro, former president of Princeton University and the University of Michigan, wrote, "Let me focus for a moment on the willingness to take informed risks. The willingness to risk failure is an essential component of most successful initiatives. The unwillingness to face the risks of failure—or an excessive zeal to avoid all risks—is, in the end, an acceptance of mediocrity and an abdication of leadership" (p. 609).

In fact, nursing leaders who have achieved the most exceptional levels of success point to significant failures that they experienced along the way—and the ways in which these failures informed and helped drive their future success.

Ann Scott Blouin recalls two distinct setbacks or disappointments in her career: "I applied twice for CNO [chief nursing officer] positions and didn't get either of them," she says. But, she adds, "In retrospect, I'm glad I didn't! Because I would never have learned the financial skills that I learned at McNeal."

She, like other nurses we spoke with, also lost a job, which can be a very painful experience. "I briefly went to Mercy, where the CEO and my colleagues and I all lost our jobs," she says. "I was there for 3 months." At that time, she says, she received some encouragement from a mentor who said, "Ann, what could you have possibly done wrong in 3 months? You barely know your way to the boardroom. March on; do your next thing; don't worry about it."

Learning from these failures is very important, she stresses. "If you've failed, and all of us have, sit back and 2, 3, or 4 years later you can reflect on it. There are some things you can learn from that. And, you can take some level of comfort that even if you didn't get the chief nursing officer job or the chief executive officer job, or even if you get fired—which many of us have—you can learn something from it, and you can move on."

A New Type of Boss: Board, Investors, and Association Members

One of the key distinctions between line level employees and those who move up into the higher leadership ranks of an organization is the shift from generally being accountable to one individual (your supervisor or manager) to being accountable to many individuals. At the highest level of the organization, for instance, the CEO reports to a board of directors that can consist of numerous individuals, all with different priorities, backgrounds, and beliefs. Even other members of the C-suite must learn to effectively manage these multiple relationships.

Managing these multiple relationships can be challenging, to say the least, and you may not always be successful. In fact, in at least one of our experiences as a CEO with a board of individuals who represented some of the most senior leaders in health care and, in fact, in the country, it was recognized that managing the group simply was not going to happen. Despite past experience and past effectiveness in managing multiple constituents, this group just simply defied management.

That experience, you will be happy to hear, was far outside the norm, fortunately. Still, the task of managing multiple bosses is always a challenge, specifically because the personalities, goals, and focus of these individuals often vary significantly. Your challenge as you get closer to the top of the organization is to effectively manage these varying opinions and perspectives.

The key to doing that, we believe, is establishing relationships. It is critical that you really get to know all of those who represent your "bosses"—whether that means the CEO, board members, association executives, area business leaders and politicians, and even patients and staff. In truth, your "bosses" might be considered anyone whose support approval you need in order to move forward with your own agenda.

In working with C-suite executive and board members, we have found that the key priority is attempting to reach consensus around some reasonable, measurable outcomes that you intend to achieve over time. Working together, you want to identify what success will look like 1, 2, or 3 years or more from now. Clarify that desired outcome, agree to it, and then let that be your focus as you address whatever myriad issues come before you. So, maybe it is having more members in your association, maybe it is having better clinical outcomes, maybe it is achieving some revenue goal. Whatever it is, get it out on the table, get everyone focused on that single goal, and refer back to that goal whenever you may be at a crossroads.

Connie serves on a university board where the vision focuses on improving the quality of students and student outcomes in terms of getting jobs and, aligned with improving the quality of students, improving faculty recruitment. As long as all of our board members are focused on this core vision, we can have discussions that might be contentious at times, but that will ultimately be settled based on a solid understanding of what we are all about. Importantly, you need to keep the main thing *the main thing*. And, you need to ensure that those who surround you know what the main thing is, agree that it is the main thing, and work together to achieve that main thing. Not easy to do, but that focus can help relieve a great deal of the angst and stress of trying to wrangle with multiple individuals from multiple backgrounds and with multiple individual beliefs.

Leadership is about ambiguity and, certainly, as nurses in leadership roles seek to navigate the many relationships they will be involved with, they will encounter ambiguity. It can be difficult to fully realize what challenges these ambiguities actually represent until you have "been there, done that," but in 1994, when reflecting on his classic 1974 article "Skills of an Effective Administrator," Robert L. Katz acknowledged that he "took too simplistic and naïve a view of the chief executive's role" (*Harvard Business Review*, 1998, p. 10). He went on to say, "My extensive work with company presidents and my own personal experience as a chief executive have given me much more respect for the difficulties and complexities of that role. I now know that every important executive action must strike a balance among so many conflicting values, objectives and criteria that it will *always* be suboptimal from any single viewpoint. *Every* decision or choice affecting the whole enterprise has negative consequences for some of the parts" (*Harvard Business Review*, 1998, p. 10).

It is a valid perspective and an accurate assessment of the unique challenges that C-level positions hold for their incumbents. A key way that leaders attempt to navigate this tricky terrain is by seeking to understand the viewpoints, perspectives, values, and needs of the various constituents they serve.

Understanding Your Constituents

Leaders have multiple constituents. In fact, the greater your leadership role, the more constituents you will have. Consider, for instance, President Obama's constituents compared with the constituents that your hospital CEO might have, or the constituents of the president of your state association. The bigger and broader your reach, the more individuals you will need to interact with and, at times, appease. Clearly that can become a challenge.

A key factor in working effectively with the constituents you serve is understanding their needs, interests, and desires. And, importantly, understanding what they expect from you. What is the most important role you play with them?

The first morning that Connie arrived at the University of San Francisco to serve as associate dean, she met with the dean, a nun, who took her on a tour. On their walk, she pointed out the University of California-San Francisco and said, "Look over there. That's a very good school, and it's a very cheap school. Students there pay very low tuition. They teach nursing, and they teach medicine." Then, she turned her attention to their school and said, "We are Jesuit; we are Catholic; we are very expensive. Parents make enormous sacrifices to send their children to this school, and they often have several children they send here." Most importantly, she made this point: "We don't teach nursing here. We teach Susan, and we teach John, and we teach Chris. The best professors remember that it is all about the students. It's not about nursing, and it's not about USF. It's about helping the students achieve their goals."

In her role as dean, she was singularly focused on the students. She had four large Rolodexes on her desk that contained details on her students—their photos, where they went to high school, siblings and parents who attended the school. While she was on phone calls, she would go through these Rolodexes and commit the information to memory. Later, when she encountered students, she could refer to them by name and refer to bits and pieces about them and their families that she recalled. She made the main thing *the main thing*.

That is what leaders must remember. You have to keep the main thing *the main thing*. You set the example. You are on display, and people are watching you. If you do not demonstrate a clear focus on your constituents and a real desire to meet their needs, you cannot expect your faculty, your nurses, or your staff members to do so. You must be a leader who leads with integrity. Your reputation is everything.

Executive Leadership Lessons

- There is a national call for nurses to have more influence. There has never been a better time for you to leverage these opportunities to achieve your personal and professional goals.

- Start along your path to the corner office through early leadership experiences. Take advantage of opportunities to serve through volunteer involvement or other organizations you are involved with.

- Career disappointments are part of the journey and something you should expect and be prepared for. What is important is how you deal with, and learn from, those disappointments.

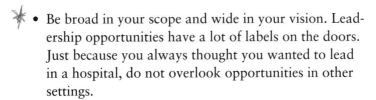

- Be broad in your scope and wide in your vision. Leadership opportunities have a lot of labels on the doors. Just because you always thought you wanted to lead in a hospital, do not overlook opportunities in other settings.

- You should spend more time exploiting your strengths than whining about your weaknesses.

- You have to know money; you have to be financially literate in the culture you want to move ahead in and understand how finances drive your organization's success.

- Although the path to the top is often circuitous, it provides opportunities for unique learning.

- As you move higher up in the organization, the complexity and multiplicity of relationships increase. You need to be prepared to navigate this increasing complexity.

- Respect is reciprocal. You have to show respect for others in the way you act, behave, and live your life if you expect them to respect you back.

References

American Association of Nurse Executives (AONE). (2005). AONE nurse executive competencies. *Nurse Leader, 3*(1), 15-22.

DePree, Max. (1989). *Leadership is an art.* New York, NY: Doubleday Business.

Harvard Business Review. (1998). *Business classics: Fifteen key concepts for managerial success.* Boston, MA: Harvard Business School Press Books. (Reprinted from Katz, Robert L. (1974). Skills of an effective administrator. *Harvard Business Review, 52*(5), 90-102.)

Health Resources and Services Administration. (2004, March). *The registered nurse population: Findings from the March 2004 National Sample Survey of Registered Nurses.* Retrieved from http://bhpr.hrsa/gav/healthworkforce/rnsurveys/rnsurvey2004.pdf

Helgesen, S. (1995). *The female advantage.* New York, NY: Doubleday Currency.

Institute of Medicine (IOM). (2010). *The future of nursing: Leading change, advancing change.* Washington, DC, National Academies Press.

Mann, E. (1949). The head nurse as a leader. *American Journal of Nursing, 49*(10), 626-628.

McDonagh, K., & Paris, N. (2012). The leadership labyrinth: Career advancement for women. *Frontiers of Health Services Management, 28*(4), 22-28.

MinorityNurse.com. (2012). Nursing statistics. Retrieved from http://www.minoritynurse.com/minority-nursing-statistics

Rath, T., & Conchie, B. (2009). *Strengths-based leadership.* Washington, DC: Gallup Press.

Robert Wood Johnson Foundation. (2010). Groundbreaking new survey finds that diverse opinion leaders say nurses should have more influence on health systems and services. Retrieved from http://www.rwjf.org/content/rwjf/en/about-rwjf/newsroom/newsroom-content/2010/01/groundbreaking-new-survey-finds-that-diverse-opinion-leaders-say.html

Robert Wood Johnson Foundation. (2011). Memo to aspiring nurse executive and leaders: "This is your time!" Retrieved from http://www.rwjf.org/en/about-rwjf/newsroom/newsroom-content/2011/06/memo-to-aspiring-nurse-executives-and-leaders-this-is-your-time.html

Shapiro, H. T. (1990). The willingness to risk failure. *Science, 250*(4981), 609.

Chapter 2

Leveraging Your Passionate Mission and Your Valuable Intellectual Capital

"In early 2011, high above Park Avenue in midtown Manhattan, a meeting took place in the well-appointed offices of a publicly traded investment banking firm. This $6.5 billion private equity firm makes large investments in health care-related enterprises, including hospital systems. The banker hosting the meeting described the company's investment strategy and interest in the health care sector, stating that, 'Given the population demographics and looming government reform initiatives, our company is interested in making investments in successful health care organizations and leveraging our investment to make their performance even stronger. We understand that value in health care is not measured by profit alone but by

clinical outcomes as well.' He further stated that the 'one area we have yet to figure out is nursing. We know that nursing is the key to making these organizations efficient, but we can't find qualified nurses financially savvy enough to manage our operations and provide us investment guidance. My partners and I think nurses are the ones with the cost/quality knowhow. Do you realize how valuable your intellectual capital is to Wall Street? Do you realize that today, Wall Street investors would pay substantially for nurses with these business skills? We need you to advise us on managing our investments and providing value in this sector.'"

–True story, Therese Fitzpatrick, April 1, 2011

Understanding the Big Picture

What an exciting time to be a nurse leader. Over the course of our careers, many of us have lamented that we have been underappreciated by our organization's senior leaders and marginalized in the larger dialogue focused on shaping the future of health care. After all, we represent the voice of the consumer at these important strategic tables, right? Right? Aren't we the discipline with the expertise in coordinating care, managing clinical outcomes, running complex organizations, and serving as patient navigators through the turbulent waters of contemporary health care? Is this the opportunity we have been dreaming about—finally, a seat at the power table? But are we ready? How do we package and communicate our substantial expertise in a manner that demonstrates that executive nurses are the source of leadership for critical policy decisions and at the most strategic levels of businesses and health care organizations? We are increasingly being calling upon by unexpected audiences with rapidly expanding needs for our perspectives, leadership, and strategic vision.

I excitedly spoke with several colleagues after this Wall Street meeting, asking whom we might know that would be interested in such an exciting opportunity. After all, this would be the perfect role for the business-savvy chief nursing executive. Talk about the corner office—it does not get bigger than this, or so I thought. Yet those niggling feelings of insecurity began to surface during the course of these conversations, those age-old insecurities about our abilities and self-perceptions and business knowhow. "What intellectual capital do I possess that investors might find valuable?" "I know how to talk with my C-suite colleagues, but can I use those same skills with investors?" "How do I know how to valuate this intellectual capital you claim I possess?"

What Is Intellectual Capital?

As your guides to the corner office, we are suggesting that the call to action is one of articulating our intellectual capital (IC) and repurposing this valuable commodity for the larger business community. As health care leaders, we have the requisite skills to invite ourselves to the table, but as our corner office executive nurses contend, we need to walk tall and demonstrate the confidence that emanates from our capabilities. Now is *not* the time to impose our own glass ceiling on nurse leaders with the interest, aptitude, and tenacity to enter uncharted territory, whether that be a well-deserved seat in the corner office, Wall Street, the State House, at the highest levels of our military, or as an entrepreneur. Rhonda Anderson agrees: "One of the most pivotal things and something I would suggest is that people really need to be aware of not waiting for those things to be coming at them, but always scanning the universe in our industry as well as nonindustry areas, because the other areas drive what our industry does, meaning the benefit purchasers drive what we need to be doing in terms of giving value to them and their members."

Perhaps the best place to begin the conversation is by defining and understanding the notion of IC. What is it that Wall Street investors and other industry leaders find so captivating and necessary to their business strategies? Covell (2008) suggests that understanding nursing IC is important in the larger dialogue of health care, specifically, the influence of nurses' knowledge, skills, and experience on clinical and organizational outcomes. Edvinsson and Malone (1997) created the model for IC, stating that human capital is the primary concept of IC theory, which is widely defined as the organization's intangible assets of knowledge, skills, and the experience of employees. Human capital resides with the employee and is therefore not owned by the organization, but rather is loaned to the organization by the employee and leaves the organization when the employee leaves (Stewart, 1997). Employers make an investment in human capital resources by hiring people with the knowledge, talent, and experience to perform their jobs well (Covell, 2008).

Not long ago, when we lived in the Industrial Age, our economy was centered on machine-based manufacturing and the transit of those goods and products across the country, and eventually the globe. During this era, the assets of a business were tangible: real property, inventory, and equipment. When assigning a monetary value to a company, it was relatively easy: A dollar value could be allocated to the tangible assets, which was added to the revenue earned through the sale of products—in other words, the value according to the balance sheet. This is often referred to as the book value of an enterprise. In this conventional wisdom, however, the true value of a company is what the market is willing to pay. As we have recently experienced with the housing crisis, a beautiful home worth $500,000 may only sell for $350,000 if that is all that the market is willing to pay. Frustrating to the seller, no doubt, the market forces favor the buyer in this instance. Conversely, however, depending on the industry as well as the market forces, a buyer may be willing to pay significantly more than the book value of a company, or what is referred to as "multiples" of the book value.

This is every entrepreneur's dream: to create a company of such value and so much potential that a buyer is willing to pay more than book value.

But we know that companies have more value than the machines on the shop floor or the desks in their offices. Is the value of McDonald's based solely on its inventory of food preparation equipment? Or did Apple become the most valuable company in history based on the real estate value of its Cupertino, California, corporate headquarters? Factors such as customer relationships and marketing strategies significantly contribute to the success of any business. One's ability to grow a company's revenues is based on creating new markets for the sale of goods and services or through selling more of a company's product to existing customers. This is often referred to as organic growth. "Organic growth in business suggests that a company is expanding its business through the use of its own resources and assets. Growing organically means a company expands without the use of mergers and acquisitions or other takeovers. An emphasis on organic growth is valued by many executives and investors since it shows a long-term, solid commitment to building the business" (eHow.com, 2012).

These "softer" attributes, intangible assets, are often referred to as goodwill. It represents the measure of the value of the organization that goes beyond its specific physical assets. This includes good relationships with suppliers and customers, a favorable reputation for high quality, and other similar values that are difficult to quantify. Although most organizations have goodwill, they usually do not show it on the financial statement because of the difficulty in assigning a value. It will appear on a financial statement when an organization is purchased, particularly if the purchaser paid more than the value of the tangible assets. The accountants will assume that the excess payment was for general goodwill of the company (Finkler, Jones, & Kovner, 2013).

IC in a Knowledge Economy

But we are no longer living in an age characterized by heavy manufacturing and assembly lines, and when human resources were considered expenses. Manufacturing companies during the Industrial Age grew in size and profits by improving their engineering efficiency, leading to faster production cycles and greater output. In the present day, information represents the new raw material. There has emerged a new economic order resulting from the management of this new raw material, in which intangible assets, while supporting the main source of value creation, have assumed a preponderant role. In accounting these materials are known as intangibles, in economic theory as knowledge assets, and in management theory as IC. And while its essence represents an asset without physical existence, it is the foundation upon which contemporary enterprises are built, innovation occurs, and wealth is created (Madhulika & Vivek, 2010).

In a knowledge economy, there is a significantly greater reliance on human ideas, services, and information technology than in production-oriented industries. In order to become market leaders, employers must value employees as assets, especially if those employees know how to navigate information sources and use the knowledge to contribute to the company's bottom line (Kamberg, 2007). In fact, the evidence now demonstrates that intangible assets are the main source of value creation in the new economic order. The impact of knowledge capital investment on gross domestic product surpassed for the period 1991–2000 that of fixed capital investment (Madhulika & Vivek, 2010). In other words, for the first time in history the knowledge and experience employees bring to their employers are substantially more valuable in the creation of wealth than the physical assets of our nation's businesses.

The English philosopher Francis Bacon (n.d.) once declared that "knowledge is power." Management scholars have firmly established the role of knowledge as a key competitive resource and further acknowledge the importance of knowledge in strategic and competitive organizational contexts. Knowledge is arguably *the* strategic resource, and companies supersede in markets by their ability to create and harness this valuable human resource (Nag & Gioia, 2012).

IC *Is* the Competitive Advantage

Kaplan and Norton (2004b, 2006) have written extensively about the critical importance of developing human capital—the intangible asset—in an effort to support the strategic imperatives of the enterprise but also to spark innovation. They contend that three categories of intangible assets are essential for implementing any strategy: human capital, where the intellectual wherewithal of the enterprise resides; information capital; and organizational capital, which includes the culture, mission, and leadership strength of the enterprise (Kaplan & Norton, 2004a).

"Sustaining competitive advantage requires that organizations continually innovate to create new products, services, and processes. Successful innovation drives customer acquisition and growth, margin enhancement, and customer loyalty. Without innovation, a company's value proposition can eventually be imitated, leading to competition solely on price for its now commoditized products and services" (Kaplan & Norton, 2004b, p. 135). In fact, their creation of the Balanced Scorecard as a framework for describing strategies for creating value within an organization has, as a primary tenet, the learning and growth of human capital as a lead indicator for internal process, customer, and financial performance (Kaplan & Norton, 2004b). This suggests that organizational knowledge is substantially created through acquiring knowledgeable individual talent and creating an organizational environment predicated on learning and synergy as a means of creating collective (group or organizational) knowledge.

Weston, Estrada, and Carrington (2007) suggest that IC is not limited to having knowledgeable workers in isolation, but the knowledge of the employees becomes an asset when it is utilized, shared, and expressed in the organization. "Maximizing intellectual capital of individuals, leaders, and teams without simultaneously creating a culture and infrastructure that translates this wisdom into intellectual and performance gain for the organization is not a good investment. Rather, it is like acquiring and investing in new buildings and equipment without having a plan for leveraging physical capital into new programs, customers or revenue" (Weston et al., 2007, p. 7).

Phillips and Phillips (2002) offer a model for IC that describes the various categories and ubiquitous nature of this intangible asset within an organization. While developed primarily as a means of quantifying IC for accounting purposes, the model, when situated within the context of a health care enterprise, can be employed by the executive nurse in understanding and managing the pervasive influence of IC in every aspect of an enterprise, from how customer relationships are managed to the inspirational impact of IC on research and development activities. As noted in Figure 2.1, IC theory proposes relationships among human capital, informational capital, and organizational capital as a means of improving business outcomes.

This intangible asset model can also serve as a foundation for describing and monetizing our executive IC as we describe our value proposition to internal as well as external audiences. Our executive nursing IC impacts each of these critical organizational factors. Our expertise and dynamic influence are felt in the manner in which we bring value to our customers, in the creation of organizational intelligence around our services and products, and in the creation of a learning organization. Arguably, the areas where we provide tremendous value, which have not yet been fully articulated, are around innovation and research and development, for example, care models, inventions, and evidence-based protocols.

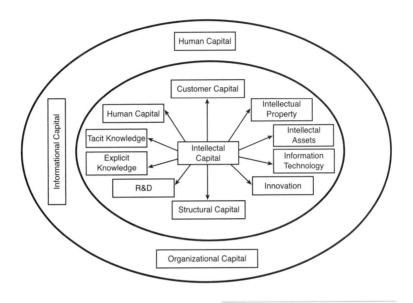

FIGURE 2.1

Intellectual Capital Model

Knowledge Is Power: What Is Our Nursing IC, and How Do We Value and Leverage It?

It is easy to make the case that executive nurses possess the requisite competencies, knowledge, and experience that provide a strategic advantage for a variety of enterprises and industries with an interest in health care: the insurance industry, large health systems, the military, and regulatory agencies, to name a few. Our proficiency and experience with patients as well as the inefficient systems and processes that often plague the health care industry also make us creative inventors and entrepreneurs, as we look for new and different opportunities to fulfill our mission to improve the lives and well-being of the members of our communities or patients within the health care system. We are notorious "fixers" with an astounding ability to move mountains and, oftentimes, entrenched systems if it means an improvement in the lives and well-being of our patients or employees. Pat O'Donoghue stated this point quite aptly while reflecting on her own career: "There are several experiences that I think were important to me. One occurred in the emergency department when I started, so very long ago. I came to realize that I was a competent nurse; I was a good nurse. And from that came a self-confidence that has served me well from those early days. I believe strongly that in order to succeed, you have to be self-confident, and that comes from being competent in what you do. Nursing was the first place where I gained that confidence based on competence."

Leveraging That Nursing Know-How

Executive nurses who aspire to lead organizations or otherwise hold positions of great public trust, such as political office or in regulatory agencies, will often report that they view these roles as an extension of their commitment to care for people or to educate others to care for people. They have acquired the skills and experiences to create an environment that supports a culture of caring and clinical expertise at the most senior levels of the enterprise and to drive these values throughout the entire organization. Because executive nurses understand and have lived the experience at the level at which services are provided, they have a clear vision of systems and processes that will provide value to the employees who interact directly with the customer, thereby improving experiential and clinical outcomes. The executive nurse also appreciates the fact that the best outcomes do not occur by serendipity but rather through the creation of healthy business environments. Only in a flourishing organization can the best talent be hired and investments in this talent along with the physical plant can be made. The implementation of best practices leading to optimal outcomes, whether clinical or business, requires sufficient structural and relationship capital to create an environment of collaboration with both internal as well as external stakeholders. In order to achieve this, an organization must be financially and strategically healthy.

Successful executive nurses do not view cost and quality as opposite sides of a coin but rather in a value-based context. In applied economic terms, this is referred to as *utility*, or the benefit gained by a consumer from the purchase of goods or services. The more benefit gained, the greater utility. Marginal utility suggests that there is a tipping point whereby the additional costs do not necessarily produce a significantly greater outcome- or utility (Finkler et al., 2013). An executive nurse possesses the business and management proficiency to determine that critical tipping point and, furthermore, execute the precise strategy to lead the organization toward that outcome. It is not a matter of simply "throwing" additional human and financial capital at a problem, particularly in an era of fiscal constraint. The sophisticated executive understands the most effective allocation of resources as well as the point at which an additional investment would not necessarily lead to additional benefit. It might be argued that the executive dexterity to manage financial risk/benefit is perhaps one of the most critical competencies in this knowledge-based business economy, where IC investment substantially drives the profit and therefore the success of the organization.

This work is not for the faint of heart, since it requires significant analytical, execution, and communication skills. We have a unique ability and, arguably, responsibility to interpret the value we are providing to the consumer and to direct the investment of resources to the greatest benefit. This difficult job cannot be performed in isolation but rather through collaboration. In fact, expert leaders view their role expansively, articulating their position as leader of the enterprise and not simply the nursing organization. This is a professional imperative if one aspires to break into a senior executive role: It is incumbent upon the leader to leverage all IC within the organization in the execution of the strategy. Expanding our understanding and interprofessional empathy requires a greatly enhanced worldview and deeper understanding of capabilities and issues confronting all professional disciplines within the enterprise.

A consistent theme emerged from our conversations with the corner office executive nurses: As they established their careers, they developed the ability to describe their capabilities in terms of the value they would bring to a business enterprise, whether that was in the role of CEO, running for political office, or selling a business concept to a group of investors. No matter the circumstance, these successful leaders took complete responsibility for their careers and strategically garnered the requisite education and varied experiences to create opportunities for themselves, demonstrating that they could add value in myriad ways and often in groundbreaking positions not traditionally held by nurses.

They learned to identify, describe, and leverage their IC— their nursing know-how: the knowledge, skills, and experience generated over rich and fulfilling careers—and communicate this expertise to potential employers or other constituents in order not only to enhance their personal circumstances but also to advance their passionate vision for professional nursing. The secret is in quantifying and describing this intangible but important asset and marketing these capabilities to diverse audiences within the health care and business communities. This process need not be intimidating or difficult; our clinical assessment and implementation expertise can be easily repurposed with this new goal in mind. In fact, our corner office executives reported that the nursing or scientific process that served them well as the foundation of their clinical experiences assumed a new level of importance when applied to leveraging their personal IC.

The ability to assess and diagnose, plan, execute, and evaluate assumes a new dimension when applied to the business environment. Rather than assessing individual patients or communities, business leaders assess the economic environment or an investment opportunity or even the political landscape in preparation for a run for office. In lieu of vital signs and a pertinent medical history, business leaders are assessing the external economic and regulatory forces confronting their enterprise. They may need to determine if there is a market for their particular service or product and how much that market might be willing to pay. Are there tax implications that must be considered when deciding on a particular corporate structure based on projected earnings? Similar to the importance of a thorough assessment and well-thought-out plan in the delivery of nursing care to a patient, the execution of a business strategy is less risky and significantly easier to measure and monitor when it is the result of comprehensive planning. In addition to an environmental, financial, and legal assessment of a particular business opportunity, the leader must possess the requisite professional repertoire of skills.

The Nursing Process Serves Us Well

Each of the corner office executives referenced the nursing process as an important and valuable methodology for executive problem-solving. Pat O'Donoghue perhaps said it best: "As you can see, I have had many unique experiences, and in each of them, I have drawn from nursing. I have been a senior administrator in four institutions of higher education, and in each, I always go back to my roots in nursing. Let me explain. I believe nursing has so much to offer to so many different disciplines. I was interviewed for my alumni magazine a couple of times. One thing I always talk about is how I continue each day to use the nursing process; I use that every day in my life in decision-making. I also learned early on what responsibility and accountability is associated with that decision-making. The confidence that nursing gives you in your direct service to patients is something that will serve you well. The fact that you have to think and plan and organize are invaluable skills wherever you find yourself. There's not one thing that I couldn't attribute to nursing that I use today. Not one thing."

Assess Your Current Capabilities

When considering a position in the corner office, it is necessary to conduct an honest and thoughtful self-assessment of one's capabilities, experience, and strengths as well as to identify those opportunities for continued development. Each of the corner office executives acknowledged the importance of finding a colleague or mentor who is brutally honest and forthcoming with performance feedback. An executive nurse who aspires to a role in the highest levels of leadership, an executive nurse must possess the ability to be introspective, to be relatively tough-skinned, and to express the willingness to accept feedback from a trusted colleague who is interested in his or her success. The trust that you place in this individual allows for the expression of honest perceptions of your strengths and weaknesses, and therefore his or her feedback becomes quite meaningful and will actually help to build self-esteem.

Whether executing a business plan as an entrepreneur or aspiring to the corner office within an enterprise, expert business skills are essential. Hisrich, Peters, and Shepherd (2008) contend that the creation of a business plan of any sort in any industry requires a specific skill set. They suggest that the businessperson or entrepreneur critically assess his or her competence in each of these areas as related to the venture or enterprise he or she is choosing to lead. The results of the self-assessment can form the basis for continuing education or in garnering additional experiences. Oftentimes it may point to the need for experts or consultants to lend their expertise to the venture, especially if time is of the essence. As difficult as it may be to admit, the goal is a successful and profitable enterprise; therefore, asking for assistance where skills and experience may be lacking is not a failure. Rather, it demonstrates a sense of self-confidence and willingness to put aside personal insecurities for the greater organizational good.

The basic business skills as outlined in the self-assessment tool created by Robert Hisrich (Hisrich et al., 2008) and shown in Table 2.1 are necessary in any type of business endeavor, whether a large complex enterprise or a one-person entrepreneurial venture where the owner is responsible for all aspects of developing, marketing, and providing a service or product. In order to stay competitive, contemporary knowledge-based organizations must demonstrate a more entrepreneurial-oriented management focus rather than the traditional administrative top-down approach. Conceptually, this suggests that the successful executive possesses a strategic orientation with an uncanny ability to identify opportunities. Instead of the traditional administrative approach of controlling resources, the entrepreneurial executive understands how and where to direct resources for the greatest return on the investment of human and other types of capital.

The world-renowned management expert Peter Drucker, in a 1988 *Harvard Business Review* commentary, expressed an opinion of leadership in the world economy that holds true in the new millennium, where knowledge is the raw material of capital production. He contends that there are seven critical elements of management—the intangible assets—that give any organization the competitive edge and increase shareholder value. Executive leaders with the skills and ability to create an organizational knowledge structure will be able to transform common knowledge into uncommon knowledge and create distinctive corporate advantages.

- Management is about human beings; therefore, the task is to make people capable of joint performance, to make strengths effective and weaknesses irrelevant.

- Management deals with the integration of people in a common venture that is deeply embedded in culture.

- Every enterprise requires simple, clear, and unifying objectives; a clear mission; and a common vision.

- It is management's role to create a learning and teaching organization.

- Every enterprise is composed of individuals with different skills and knowledge; therefore, it is incumbent upon us to build systems of communication and responsibility.

- Market standing, innovation, productivity, quality, people development, and financial results are all critical to a company's survival.

- The result of a business is a satisfied customer; therefore, there are no results within its walls.

(Drucker, 1988, pp. 75-76)

Executive nurses possess the knowledge and capabilities to sit in the most strategic positions within today's most complex and confounding organizations. As a strategic source of IC, we bring not only the individual skills to excel in meeting customer needs but also to create the environment to leverage the IC of all constituents, whether they be employees and other professionals or the communities our businesses serve. Those who are in a position to invest in growing organizations or boards of companies, and health care organizations searching for leaders with the ability to create value for stakeholders, recognize that executive nurses have those requisite skills and will, in increasing numbers, invite them to take their hard-earned seat in the corner office.

Therese can attest to this through personal experience: "In my business, I have an opportunity to interface with investors a fair amount—folks who are investing private equity, Wall Street firms that are investing in health care systems. When I meet with these Wall Street guys, they say, 'We wish we could find nurses who understand finance and could hire them to advise us and help us understand nursing and health care.' I believe we need to harness our intellectual capital in this profession. We bring so much to the table, and I look at nurse executives and the pivotal role that they play in being able to translate patient care, patient outcomes, quality—what's important to value-based health care—and we have an opportunity to translate that not just to the rest of the world, but to the financial community as well. We have the intellectual capital that can be advising and directing on the policy side as well."

TABLE 2.1 Skills Assessment

SKILLS	EXCELLENT	GOOD	FAIR	POOR	REMEDIATION PLAN
Accounting and taxes				X	
Planning	X				
Forecasting		X			
Market research				X	
Sales				X	
Human resource management	X				
Product design		X			
Legal issues				X	
Organizing	X				

From Hisrich et al., 2008

Executive Leadership Lessons

- Be secure in the value you bring to an organization.

- Learn to articulate and value your IC; understand that it is worth a great deal in the market, and you should be compensated well for your IC.

- Become an expert in complex process analysis and improvement.

- Begin to understand risk management—not clinical risk, but rather financial and strategic risk.

- Begin to view your current role more expansively; if you are currently leading a department, begin to learn about the bigger picture; request assignments or projects that have a significant financial component or cut across the wider organization or components of the care continuum.

- Conduct an honest self-assessment; specifically, address your skill level in the basic business skills required in the corner office, and elicit feedback from a colleague who can be open and honest with you.

- Learn to use consultants—it is not possible for you to be an expert in everything, and often the organization will benefit from the opinions of an expert. Realize that it is not an indictment of your leadership or individual expertise.

- When quantifying the value of your business, remember the importance of goodwill and the value of relationships and reputation.

- Learn to value the expertise your staff brings to the enterprise; this is the real wealth in a knowledge economy.

References

Bacon, F. (n.d.). Retrieved from http://www.brainyquote.com/quotes/authors/f/francis_bacon.html

Covell, C. L. (2008). The middle-range theory of nursing intellectual capital. *Journal of Advanced Nursing, 63*(1), 94-103.

Drucker, P. F. (1988). Management and the world's work. *Harvard Business Review, 66*(5), 65-76.

Edvinsson, L., & Malone, M. S. (1997). *Intellectual capital: Realizing your company's true value by finding its hidden brainpower.* New York, NY: Harper Business Press.

eHow.com. (2012). *What is organic growth in business?* Retrieved from http://www.ehow.com/about_5059362_organic-growth-business.html

Finkler, S. A., Jones, C. B., & Kovner, C. T. (2013). *Financial management for nurse managers and executives.* St. Louis, MO: Elsevier.

Hisrich, R. D., Peters, M. P., & Shepherd, D. A. (2008). *Entrepreneurship.* Boston, MA: McGraw-Hill Irwin.

Kamberg, M. L. (2007). The knowledge economy is here: Are you ready? *Women in Business, 59*(2), 13-17.

Kaplan, R. S., & Norton, D. P. (2004a). Measuring the strategic readiness of intangible assets. *Harvard Business Review, 7*(2), 52-63.

Kaplan, R. S., & Norton, D. P. (2004b). *Strategy maps: Converting intangible assets into tangible outcomes.* Boston, MA: Harvard Business School Press.

Kaplan, R. S., & Norton, D. P. (2006). *Alignment.* Boston, MA: Harvard Business School Press.

Madhulika, P., & Vivek, K. (2010). The emerging business models in the knowledge economy: Its impact on society and government. *Advances in Management, 3*(8), 23-31.

Nag, R., & Gioia, D. A. (2012). From common to uncommon knowledge: Foundations of firm-specific use of knowledge as a resource. *Academy of Management Journal, 55*(2), 421-457.

Phillips, J. J., & Phillips, P. P. (2002). Measuring and monitoring intellectual capital: Progress and future challenges. In P. P. Phillips (Ed.), *Measuring intellectual capital.* Alexandria, VA: ASTD Press.

Stewart, T. (1997). *Intellectual capital: The new wealth of organizations.* New York, NY: Currency Doubleday.

Weston, M., Estrada, N. A., & Carrington, J. (2007). Reaping benefits from intellectual capital. *Nursing Administration Quarterly, 31*(1), 6-12.

Chapter 3

Becoming an Entrepreneur: Harnessing Your Creativity

"Being a great CEO requires having great discipline. It takes thought and discipline to be able to make sure my compass is pointed in a direction where I can be most creative to the biggest need and to restructure what needs to be restructured—for me to do that in a way that doesn't prevent the people around me from achieving their goals."

–P. K. Scheerle, September 2012

A tornado was the impetus for Connie's entry into the nursing profession. "I initially went into nursing, if truth be told, because we had a tornado in my little Wisconsin town, and the first people who got through to help us and help the people in the town were nurses," she recalls. "They were driving a Red Cross truck and they did everything from start blood and give immunizations to help extricate people from buildings. They physically pulled people out of buildings and served coffee and donuts. I just thought it was incredibly wonderful that these women in these white dresses and red capes driving these trucks with red crosses on them could save lives like that and help people, and it just seemed very exciting to me and very dramatic to me.

"I saw those nurses and began getting very interested in nursing. I went to the public library and began reading every book I could get my hands on—I read about Sue Barton and other nurses; I read about army nurses, detective nurses, pilot nurses, you name it. I just thought it was incredibly interesting."

Her interest led to a decision to volunteer at a local hospital; later she became president of student nurses and pursued her nursing degree through the University of Wisconsin. Her career has spanned clinical nursing, education, administration, and entrepreneurialism. She views her career not as a pathway but more of a "strong commitment to making things better for patients and for caregivers." She says, "I just had this mission that I wanted things to be better for patients, and I wanted things to be better for the people who took care of them."

Initially, she says, that meant being a good staff nurse. But then she began to see the value of academics—of teaching other nurses how to do good things. While in academics, she worked her way up to a position as dean. Then, she says, she began to feel that academia was not close enough to patients. So, she left academia and took a position as chief nurse at Montefiore Medical Center in New York City. "In those days, Montefiore was the largest private hospital in the United States, with 2,500 registered nurses and 10,000 other employees who worked for me," she says. "It was an opportunity to have an impact again—both on the patients and on the staff, and also, for me, it was an opportunity to define new roles for nursing that I had never thought about."

While working at Montefiore, Connie worked with her boss and Mayor Ed Koch to place nurses and doctors into all of the prisons of New York City. "We had 10,000 prisoners on Rikers Island, and we were able to convince Mayor Koch that when a prisoner was sick, he was a patient and he should be cared for by people who reported to a hospital—not doctors and nurses who worked for a warden," she recalls. "We were able to do things like that at Montefiore—we were able to sort of reimagine and redefine where nurses could work and what they could do and who our patients were." They were not just in hospitals. They were also in prisons. They were in their homes. The experience, she says, shaped her vision of how nurses could make an impact and how she could help them do so.

Connie left Montefiore to come back to the Midwest to take a position as vice president for the American Hospital Association (AHA); it was her first foray outside the world of academic health centers. "When I got to the AHA, I realized that most hospitals have fewer than 100 beds," she says. "Most hospitals have nurses who have to do two or three kinds of patient care. Most hospitals have nurses who know most of the patients and their families." Her experience there involved research into the labor market—why nurses worked and what it would take to get them to work more. "I had these 5,500 hospitals that were members and could really take a look at differences from hospital to hospital and start identifying best practices," she says. That experience served as the launching point for her entry into the private sector and her entrepreneurial efforts to "make things better in a broad-based way through consulting."

P. K. Scheerle has also made a career as an entrepreneur. She founded American Nursing Services, Inc., in 1982, built the company up to 28 locations, and sold it in 2002. Today she is an owner of Gifted Nurses, a private, in-home care and staff relief service that has been in service since 2006. Like many entrepreneurs, *being* an entrepreneur is in her blood—it is who she is.

Roy Simpson considers himself to be more of an "intrapreneur"—someone who works in an entrepreneurial mode within an organization. He says, "I think I do better in an intrapreneurial world, not necessarily an entrepreneurial world, where the founders understand entrepreneurship—because they are open for new business entities, and when you do a merger and acquisition, it's based on sound principles. I think that that's one thing that nurses don't realize, that in order to grow the profession of nursing, we could really apply these same principles to our professional organizations, and we could look at mergers and acquisitions. We will never do well with 500 of us in different organizations, but we may do better if we looked at mergers and acquisitions. I mean, we still have companies that keep some of their tenets to what they were ascribed to, but they're under different holding companies. I think we need to look at this business model professionally in order to be able to survive the future."

The Entrepreneurial Mind-set

We know that health care reform represents challenges and risk to health care organizations and practitioners. Importantly, though, reform also creates many opportunities for nurses who are poised to take on new leadership roles within and outside of health care organizations.

In *The Future of Nursing* report, the Robert Wood Johnson Foundation indicated that nurses were in a position to play a vital role in helping to realize objectives to make health care accessible, acceptable, and affordable, but that, in order to make this happen, certain barriers would need to be addressed. These barriers, according to the report, include "nurses' inability to practice to their full extent, lack of access to an education system that allows for seamless progression to higher levels, and lack of opportunity for full partnership with other professionals. Other needs are improved research, better data collection, and information infrastructure on health care workforce requirements" (Institute of Medicine [IOM], 2010, p. 1).

Wilson, Whitaker, and Whitford (2012) point out that while nurses make up the greatest proportion of the health care workforce (up to 80%), they have yet to be represented in corresponding numbers in roles that contribute in significant ways to health care challenges. They point out how emerging and evolving entrepreneurial and intrapreneurial roles in nursing are arising to meet the challenges of health care reform. This distinction is important because it recognizes the fact that nurses have the ability to serve in innovative roles *within* their organizations, as *intrapreneurs,* a term that means "a person within a large corporation who takes direct responsibility for turning an idea into a profitable finished product through assertive risk-taking and innovation" (*American Heritage Dictionary,* 2009)—basically, the same concept as the term *entrepreneur,* but within the organization.

Wilson et al. (2012) point to several characteristics that are shared by individuals in either of these roles, which include self-confidence, courage, integrity, self-discipline, and the ability to take risks, deal with failure, and articulate their goals. They recommend strategies to help promote entre- and intrapreneurship in nursing, which include:

- Nurse education that includes placement with a nurse entrepreneur or a business course to ensure that graduating nurses learn skills to lead, challenge, and be innovative

- Interdisciplinary learning so that allied health and medical professionals are introduced to the concept of nurses as equal partners in health care

- Greater opportunities for shared interdisciplinary collaboration in research, education, and practice to foster cohesion and role familiarity among health professionals

There is certainly growing recognition that organizations, particularly health care organizations, must focus on developing the competencies of intrapreneurs—the individuals who can drive innovation within an organization.

Covin and Wales (2011) explore how the concept of entrepreneurial orientation (EO) has been portrayed and assessed in prior research. They focus on four models that have been used to assess EO from an organizational standpoint:

- The Miller/Covin and Slevin (1989) EO scale

- An alternative first-order reflective EO scale corresponding to Miller's (1983) composite view of EO

- The Hughes and Morgan (2007) EO scale

- A "Type II" second-order formative EO scale based on the item pool generated by Hughes and Morgan (2007)

These and other assessments used over the years share commonalities. We will take a look at the Hughes and Morgan scale (accompanying sidebar), since it is the most recent and draws upon prior research.

THE HUGHES AND MORGAN (2007) EO SCALE

The Hughes and Morgan (2007) scale asks users to rate a series of risk-taking items on a scale of 1 to 7 with 1 being "strongly disagree" and 7 being "strongly agree."

Risk-taking items
- *The term risk-taker is considered a positive attribute for people in our business.*
- *People in our business are encouraged to take calculated risks with new ideas.*
- *Our business emphasizes both exploration and experimentation for opportunities.*

Innovativeness items
- *We actively introduce improvements and innovations in our business.*
- *Our business is creative in its methods of operation.*
- *Our business seeks out new ways to do things.*

Proactiveness items

- *We always try to take the initiative in every situation (e.g., against competitors, in projects when working with others).*
- *We excel at identifying opportunities.*
- *We initiate actions to which other organizations respond.*

Competitive aggressiveness items

- *Our business is intensely competitive.*
- *In general, our business takes a bold or aggressive approach when competing.*
- *We try to undo and out-maneuver the competition as best as we can.*

Autonomy items

- *Employees are permitted to act and think without interference.*
- *Employees perform jobs that allow them to make and instigate changes in the way they perform their work tasks.*
- *Employees are given freedom and independence to decide on their own how to go about doing their work.*
- *Employees are given freedom to communicate without interference.*
- *Employees are given authority and responsibility to act alone if they think it to be in the best interests of the business.*
- *Employees have access to all vital information.*

Our own experiences, as well as interviews with successful nurse entrepreneurs, reveal that many of these traits and characteristics are certainly present. Some other commonalities also emerge.

One important trait is the way entrepreneurs perceive failure. As P. K. Scheerle says, "There is failure at every turn, and there is success at every turn. When you're growing a company from the ground up, there are great obstacles for every entrepreneur." But, she adds, "Successful entrepreneurs see them as opportunities, and that was the case for me."

It has often been said that the real work of an organization happens in the white spaces on the organizational chart. This is also where the intra- and entrepreneurial opportunities emerge. The early industrial titans Vanderbilt, Carnegie, Ford, and Rockefeller, and even contemporary information titans such as Steve Jobs and Bill Gates, created empires while radically changing the way business is managed—all by turning problems into opportunities. Had any of these entrepreneurs been saddled by the inevitable constraints present in any complex enterprise, they would have been reticent to experiment and take risks with the inescapable failures that could have resulted. Whether looking for ways to light homes with kerosene, connect the coasts via rail, or manage terabytes of data, these inventors and entrepreneurs shared the same competitive spirit and singular focus and recognized that trial and error would be required to create a product with tremendous market potential.

Process inefficiencies are often identified by the individuals with intimate knowledge of that process—just ask any employee, no matter the industry, what keeps him or her from getting a job done faster or with greater efficiency, and ideas will abound. This is, in fact, the way many entrepreneurs and inventors get ideas for new services or products. Trialing and testing a new idea is not without inherent failure, however, and the successful entrepreneur not only knows to expect some false starts along the way but welcomes these failures as opportunities to perfect a product or even abandon an idea prior to widespread and expensive production.

Oftentimes, no matter how good the idea or how genius the invention, unintended forces may impact the implementation, sales, or manufacture of a product or service. Economic forces often have a great deal of impact on the opportunity.

Therese experienced this first-hand when seeking venture funding for a company she co-created. "We had boot-strapped the creation of the company as well as the technology platform, which supported the solution. We would have liked to have had investment support to build the platform, but this was too soon after the dotcom bubble burst, and investors were reluctant to invest in tech start-ups. We realized that no matter how good our idea, we'd have to self-fund our initial phase and look to investors for later phases of company development.

"My partner and I did just that—we worked in other positions to support our families while creating this business; that's how much we believed in the solution. We were then able to talk with investors after we had several initial clients and a developed solution. They were able to actually see the solution in operation and even talk with other clients. The process of finding investors would have looked dramatically different were it not for the dotcom bubble burst. The important thing was that we never gave up; we identified the obstacles and found a different solution. Perhaps it took a bit longer, but we never stopped."

The bottom line, Connie stresses, is to believe in yourself and believe in your potential. "Don't underestimate your potential— don't set your targets too low. Approach yourself and your career and your contributions with wonder, and don't close the door on what your potential may be.

"Many, many people—and I've worked mostly with women and mostly with nurses—have self-limiting beliefs. They say things like, 'I could never do this because . . .,' 'I could never be president of a company, or a dean, or a multimillionaire.'"

Our message to you: You can.

Eliminate that way of thinking. Most of us really have no clue about what it is we are capable of doing. We are here to encourage you to get out there and find out. Get rid of those self-limiting beliefs and learn to be open to the many possibilities that exist for nurses with their eyes on the corner office.

How Money Works, How Markets Work, How Capital Works

We have already discussed the importance of having a solid understanding of finance if you are hoping to land a spot in the corner office. In truth, whether you are managing an organization for someone else or building your own organization, recognizing how money works, how markets work, and how capital works is critical.

As an entrepreneur, you will be faced with decisions about how you will finance your organization. You may decide, as Connie has, that you prefer to grow your organization, or organizations, on your own, which is referred to as "bootstrapping." Start-up businesses that are financed through internal cash flow are bootstrapped businesses.

Guy Kawasaki, co-founder at Garage Technology Ventures, an early-stage venture capital firm for high-technology companies, and the author of a number of books on entrepreneurship and innovation, including *The Art of the Start*, is a fan of bootstrapping. In his blog, *How to Change the World* (Kawasaki, 2006), he outlines the steps involved in successful bootstrapping:

1. **Focus on cash flow, not profitability.** "You pay bills with cash," he notes.

2. **Forecast from the bottom up.** Most entrepreneurs, he says, do the opposite.

3. **Ship, then test.** Perfect is the enemy of good enough, says Kawasaki. "When your product or service is 'good enough,' get it out because cash flows when you start shipping."

4. **Forget the "proven" team.** Hire young, cheap, and hungry people, he advises.

5. **Start as a service business.** Even if your ultimate offering will be something tangible, until that offering is developed, you can provide consulting services based on your work-in-process.

6. **Focus on function, not form.** All a chair has to do "is hold your butt," he says. "It doesn't have to look like it belongs in the Museum of Modern Art."

7. **Pick your battles.** Bootstrappers, he says, "don't fight on all fronts because they cannot afford to fight on all fronts."

8. **Understaff.** Don't staff up for what could happen.

9. **Go direct.** "The optimal number of mouths (or hands) between a bootstrapper and her customer is zero," says Kawasaki.

10. **Position against the leader.** Toyota, he notes, introduced Lexus being as as good as a Mercedes but at half the price. "A cheap iPod and poor man's Bose noise-canceling headphones" could work, too, he says.

11. **Take the "red pill"**—a reference to Neo's choice in *The Matrix*. For bootstrappers, he says, a simple calculation is what really matters: amount of cash divided by cash burn per month because this will tell you how much longer you can live."

Sometimes you hear people talk about starting a business and taking "some time off of work" to plan for that business. Connie has always had a client lined up before starting a company. "I always wanted an actual customer before I had expenses; that's really important," she says.

Success requires that you have a very good idea that you will be able to sell someone on your product or service; if you cannot sell to just one client to get you started, the chances are not good that you will be able to sell to others.

Another key point relates to staffing. There can be a tendency to be hesitant to jump into big projects until staff is in place. That can be a mistake. The truth of the matter is that if you can sell your product or service successfully, you can add staff as you move forward. Do not believe you need to have a full cadre of staff on board before you can move forward.

But bootstrapping is just one option. There are other ways you can infuse money into your organization, each with its own risks and rewards. With bootstrapping, for instance, the reward is that you are in total control—it is your money; there is no one else (aside from your customers or clients) whom you are beholden to. That changes when you take money from other sources.

Raising Capital

A variety of options are available for those looking to raise capital to finance their business.

Angel Investors and Venture Capitalists

Angel investors and venture capitalists are similar in that both provide funding to entrepreneurs to help boost their ability to create and distribute their products and services through access to additional capital. The difference is that, typically, angel investors are investing their own funds, and venture capitalists are investing the pooled funds of a group of investors.

The ABC television show *Shark Tank*, a program that provides would-be entrepreneurs the opportunity to make their dreams come true through financing from "sharks" who evaluate their ideas, has helped to make the concept of angel investors and venture capitalists more familiar to the general public and provides some insights into what these investors look for when determining whether it makes sense for them to provide funding to entrepreneurs.

What do they look for? In short, they are interested in returns on their investment. These are smart people with money, and they do not want to give their money to those who are not going to provide them some value—in the form of more money—in return. So, if you can demonstrate that your business idea is sound, that there is a market for what you have to offer, and that you can deliver a sound return on the investment required to provide your product or service, you may have a shot at some of this money. The decision-making process is really no different from what your own decision-making process should be when you are deciding whether to invest in yourself. Of course, we are all enamored of our own ideas, so we tend to have a much brighter view of our potential for success—and sometimes, thankfully, we are right. It is true, though, that angel investors and venture capitalists will be much, much more stringent in their evaluation of your ability to provide the return they are looking for.

Institutional Investors

Another category of investors is institutional investors. Institutional investors are banks, insurance companies, investment advisors, and other enterprises that invest money on behalf of others, similar to venture capitalists. In the health care industry, pharmaceutical companies and insurance companies represent opportunities for institutional funding. Through the voting rights that these types of institutional investors attain from their investment, they have the ability to exercise a certain amount of control. And, there is the rub.

Whenever you are accepting funding from outside interests, the phrase "be careful what you wish for" may also apply. While the upside of attracting the interests of these investors is that you will have money infused into your business that can help you grow and expand and do the things that you would like to do, a potential downside is loss of control.

Philanthropy

Philanthropy represents another way to achieve funding for your business. This is how associations and colleges often get money and generally represents grants that organizations apply for. For instance, Connie's first two grants were from the Henry J. Kaiser Family Foundation.

Making decisions about how you will fund your company is very personal, and we all approach it differently. Connie has never taken money from outside investors to fund the companies she has started.

It is a very personal decision and a decision that will be based both on your personal philosophy and your ultimate objectives. For instance, if your goal is to become a multimillionaire, your decisions will probably be different than if your goal is to have a personal impact on some specific market or some specific issue that you have an intense passion for. In one case, you may not be as concerned about maintaining personal control as in another. Or, your passion may drive your decision to pursue investors, because you realize you simply cannot do it on your own and you are willing to give up some control to see your vision become a reality.

It is, though, all about the money. Connie has had a great deal of experience working with venture capitalists and knows that while they will tell you that they are bringing more to the table than money—that they are bringing in personal expertise related to your business—at the end of the day, what they are bringing you is money. And what they care about is money. There is nothing wrong with that; remember, "no money, no mission."

But if you are also looking for expertise, there may be other ways to attain it. Connie, for instance, created her own board of advisors when she launched her company CurranCare. She recruited six people with different backgrounds who she thought could impact her business positively and held quarterly board meetings where she could leverage their insights and expertise to the advantage of the business. When she sold the company, they benefited financially as well. But they did not have a controlling ownership in the business. Connie says, "I knew I needed external help; I needed people who would say 'no, that's the wrong approach to take,' or 'no, that's not a good decision.' I knew I needed that help, but I didn't want to give up ownership."

Connie readily acknowledges that she is biased against seeking outside funding that requires giving up control, but that she sees the value in that for others. The notion of maintaining control of your company while bringing in investment capital cannot be underestimated.

Therese notes, "The company is no longer your own when you have investors. When people give you large sums of money, they obviously have a vested interest in how that money is spent. Remember, you have an interest in your product or service, and they have a singular interest in making money on their investment, particularly if they represent other investors through a fund. You may have been required to give up a substantial percentage of ownership for that investment, perhaps even controlling interest. That, in essence, means that you are an employee of your own company! And, keep in mind, your investors typically do not have a similar understanding of health care; therefore, you will spend a lot of time explaining the essence of the industry and all of its challenges to financiers."

Oftentimes an entrepreneur seeks an investment to grow a company to the next level—in other words, to maximize production capacity, hire additional staff, or develop capacity in marketing and sales. You might also seek investment to acquire other companies or even competitors to grow market share or companies that provide complementary services in an effort to round out your offerings. In any case, you and your investors may decide that you do not possess the requisite skills to run the new enterprise and that it may be a better strategy to recruit a leader with a proven track record in your particular industry. The CEO of an enterprise doing a million dollars in annual sales has a different skill set from the CEO of a multinational company with $500 million in revenue. These are always difficult but necessary decisions and necessitate that you place the best interest of the company ahead of your personal wishes.

Do not be afraid to seek advice on the intricacies of investment capital, as there are certainly costs and benefits of any option. Remember that money always comes at a cost, whether that is in terms of interest tied to a conventional loan or percentage of equity awarded to an investor. What is of critical importance in deciding what route to take in growing your venture is determining where you want to be 5 or even 10 years into the future.

Successful entrepreneurs must have an exit strategy for their business. The most common exit strategies are selling the business, merging the business with another company, passing the business to another family member, or taking the company public. It is important to have an exit as part of the company's strategic plan. "At CurranCare we designed the company for an easy sale," Connie notes. "From the first dollar, we used a big four auditing firm, so there would never be a question about our financials. We had an advisory board that assisted us with strategy, our client contracts provided for transfer, etc."

The timing of the exit is dependent on a variety of factors. In the best situation, the business has reached its peak value, creating a great revenue opportunity for the owners. Some of the time, a great match appears for a merger that will create a whole that is bigger and better than the sum of its parts. In the typical business cycle, there are peaks, slumps, and plateaus. Keeping the company growing may require major changes in people, products, and finance. The owner may decide she would rather sell than start an entirely new business cycle. In other situations, a personal situation will dictate the need to sell. The owner may want to extract the capital for other reasons.

Whatever the reason, the selling of a company is a major event that includes bankers, lawyers, auditors, and a great deal of focus. "When I sold CurranCare," says Connie, "I hired the best help that I could find, and the sale demanded most of my time for at least 6 months." If the entrepreneur sells to another company or takes the company public, the executive team is often required to stay with the new owner for a significant period of time for "an earn out." The owners must choose to sell to a company that they are willing to work with during the transition. The sale of your company is not the end but the beginning of a new phase of the business and often an opportunity for you to move on to a new business.

The serial entrepreneur derives pleasure from starting, quickly growing, and selling businesses. She is always mindful of possible acquirers and keeps a watchful eye on the competitors as they look to expand their market share. The serial entrepreneur finds challenge in growing a business then moving on to the next interesting opportunity and does not necessarily see herself as personally tied to a particular company. On the other hand, there are successful entrepreneurs who have no desire to merge or acquire other companies and are satisfied to keep revenues at a level that can be managed without bringing in partners. Maintaining a watchful eye on quality and brand identity and providing personalized service may suggest a limited growth strategy. In any case, there are many investors interested in the health care sector and looking for interesting ideas and competent partners. The key is defining your long-term strategy.

Executive Leadership Lessons

- Sell—get someone to actually pay for your idea, whatever it is you think you are going to sell.

- You will learn a lot on the first project—use your first project as a pilot in learning. Be reasonable and see your first client as a learning or developmental partner.

- Start your company with an exit strategy to optimize your time, staff, and money.

- If you are going to take outside money, your investors expect a rapid return, and they expect that they are buying the right to influence and shape your company; they do not just write the check and walk away.

- You can actualize your passionate mission in a variety of settings—do not be self-limiting.

- Intrapreneurial opportunities exist in all organizations and can be a very good introduction to future entrepreneurial activity.

- Entrepreneurial behavior is reflected in a variety of characteristics, many of which are very common among nurses.

References

American Heritage Dictionary of the English Language (4th ed.) (2009). Boston, MA: Houghton Mifflin Company. Updated in 2009. Published by Houghton Mifflin Company.

Covin, J. G., & Wales, W. J. (2011). The measurement of entrepreneurial orientation. *Entrepreneurship Theory and Practice, 36*(4), 677-702.

Institute of Medicine (IOM). (2010). *The future of nursing: Leading change, advancing health.* Washington, DC: The National Academies Press.

Kawasaki, G. (2006, January 26). The art of bootstrapping [Blog post]. Retrieved from http://blog.guykawasaki.com/2006/01/the_art_of_boot.html/

Wilson, A., Whitaker, N., & Whitford, D. (2012). Rising to the challenge of health care reform with entrepreneurial and intrapreneurial nursing initiatives. *Online Journal of Issues in Nursing, 17*(2), 1. Retrieved from http://www.nursingworld.org/MainMenuCategories/ANAMarketplace/ANAPeriodicals/OJIN/TableofContents/Vol-17-2012/No2-May-2012/Rising-to-the-Challenge-of-Reform.html

Chapter 4
Learning the Language of Business

"Financial acumen—it's absolutely essential. I think many nurses operate from a social science frame of reference, and they may not understand the business side—the economics—of health care. To be a nurse leader you have to have a balanced perspective; you need to have an understanding of the P&L. You need to know how the balance sheet works versus an income statement. You need to understand product line profitability and how to achieve a return on your investments."

–Ann Scott Blouin, August 2012

As with any expedition to a foreign place, a great deal of preparation is required—familiarizing one's self with local customs, adjusting to a new currency, learning a new landscape. Assuming a new position, enjoying a promotion, or pursuing an opportunity outside of one's current comfort zone and expertise requires similar preparation. The corner office has a unique landscape, language, and culture, and passage to this destination requires not only an orientation and familiarization with the competencies required for the new position but also socialization to a new role identity.

Your Professional Identity

Chreim, Williams, and Hinings (2007) describe professional identity as an individual's self-definition as a member of a profession and the enactment of that professional role. This representation therefore gives rise to role identity—the goals, values, beliefs, norms, interaction styles, and time horizons that are typically associated with a role. The way professionals view their role identity is essential in how they interpret and perform in various work situations.

Gibson (2003) provides an interesting model for the development of professional self-concept at different stages of one's career, suggesting that as we mature professionally, our models for professional socialization adapt as well. The empirical data support the importance of role models in socializing individuals to new careers, organizations, and tasks. Career theory suggests that our development within an organization is characterized as a socialization process; as we traverse through various positions and levels of a corporation, we face ambiguities and change reminiscent of our initial entry into the professional world. Just as we did when entering health care as a new nurse graduate, we seek role models as exemplars of the professional skills and attributes we require to achieve our professional goals.

To facilitate the transition from nursing school to professional practice, we relied on preceptors and mentors to familiarize us with policies, procedures, advanced clinical skills, and the interprofessional teamwork required to provide clinical care in an overwhelmingly complex environment. But in addition to imparting this critical knowledge so important to assuring the optimal outcome for each patient in our charge, these practiced sages also taught us "the way things are done here"; in other words, they helped socialize us to both the profession of nursing as well as the particular organization. The role modeling construct combines the concept of *role,* which is defined as forms of behavior and activities associated with a position, with the concept of *modeling,* which is the psychological matching of cognitive skills and behavioral patterns between the mentor and mentee.

Early in their careers, novice professionals require two primary outcomes from a relationship with a mentor: first, how to perform tasks completely and professionally, and second, how to fit into their professional role both by matching the characteristics of the organizational culture and by earning the respect of their colleagues. Gibson's (2003) research demonstrated that, in this early developmental stage, novice professionals were apt to be assigned or seek out a generally positive role model who fit the traditional mold—a hierarchical superior with established job skills, behaviors, and attitudes that were in line with organizational convention. Gibson's findings support the notion that early-stage socialization is aimed at creating a viable self-concept and professional identity by observing and possibly emulating these significant others.

This model is adapted for the middle or later stages of one's career, when one is fully socialized into a profession and established as a competent member of an organization. It is at this stage that professionals might be asked to consider a promotional opportunity within a corporation or perhaps look to advance their career goals proximally, that is, maintain their current position but increase their reputation through additional responsibilities. As individuals mature in their professional roles, they become more competent in their abilities and confident in their professional identities, which leads them to seek a mentoring relationship focused on developing specific skills rather than inculcating personal attributes. But even technically proficient professionals must accept that in addition to learning new skills and reaffirming the effectiveness of their acquired talents and style, our turbulent work environments require a more nuanced approach to mentoring and role-modeling.

Each of the corner office executives expressed the importance of developing relationships with highly proficient and experienced mentors, trusted advisors, or coaches. While these individuals had achieved their own success in garnering a spot in the corner office, many, if not most, of these important advisors were from industries outside of health care. This important message emphasizes the fact that (a) the corner office repertoire of skills is universal in nature, and (b) learning this new set of competencies does not require the mentor to come from within health care. The skills required to lead any complex enterprise in a highly volatile market are both strategic and tactical in nature and include financial management, organizational strategy development, human capital management, negotiating strategies, and the ability to develop and maintain strategic relationships with key constituents, since the work of health care—or any business, for that matter—requires an entire symphony of contributors whose efforts must be coordinated.

Health care executives haven't cornered the market on leading complex organizations in highly regulated industries during tumultuous economic cycles defined by workforce shortages, political consternation, and internal structural anxiety. We have much to learn from leaders of government, the automobile industry, pharma, small businesses, technology, the airlines, or even the utilities.

The secret is integrating and applying these valuable lessons to the health care leadership environment or, for the entrepreneur, the next exciting business opportunity. The corner office executives gave example after example of the manner in which their careers were significantly shaped by individuals with the willingness to provide counsel, share personal experiences, and help define the risks associated with assertive and forward-looking decision-making. The tenacious executive nurses leveraged this information to generate their own opportunities with significantly greater confidence, assertiveness, and creativity. The fact that they had learned the language of business at the most strategic level cannot be understated, since this repertoire of competencies allowed them to develop as self-assured executives, which in turn served as the catalyst for breakthrough performances. They repeatedly told stories of being the first nurse in a position, the first woman in an elite business organization, or the determined entrepreneur who weathered the storm of naysayers to strike out with a new venture. Because they had become proficient in the language of this foreign land—the corner office—these leaders were not relegated to the role of observer or timid wallflower, but rather they came to the table as full participants and made contributions that often changed the direction of the enterprise or led to significant financial or strategic success.

Our Values, Our Selves

Imperative for the nurse with aspirations for an executive leadership position or the desire to begin a successful business is the requirement to learn a new set of relevant business skills and to become familiar with the social mores of the executive suite. Those values and beliefs we learned as an essential step in the process of being socialized into the profession of nursing provide the necessary foundation upon which to build the basis of an executive career. Contrary to the mistaken assumptions expressed by some nurses, we should not abandon our unique competencies and values as we gain access to the corner office, but rather we should build on our implicit values of empathy and caring, our scientific approach to decision-making and problem-solving, our collegial approach to accomplishing goals, and our ethical foundation in social justice.

These values provide a principled foundation for an executive career, a role in which the leader is called to inspire individual and organizational excellence, create a shared vision, and successfully manage change to attain the organization's strategic ends (Healthcare Leadership Alliance and the American College of Healthcare Executives, 2011). However, a number of practical competencies are required to lead and grow an organization in this complex environment, and attaining these skills will significantly contribute to the development of confidence in one's leadership abilities and positional authority, thereby gaining the trust of important constituents, inspiring creativity, and empowering others to achieve excellence. In reflecting on their own careers and the challenges they faced on their journey to the corner office, these executive nurses all reported that they benefited from additional education and mentorship in strategy development, strategic human capital management, and management of governance relationships, but most importantly the management of financial resources and the myriad regulations surrounding the actions and activities of providers, payers, and the consumers of health care.

Although they were adept at managing departmental or programmatic operating and capital budgets and even cash budgets, managing real estate investments, corporate investment strategy, multimillion or even billion-dollar profit and loss statements, and enormous capital projects required disciplined preparation. The confidence that stemmed from acquiring this expertise set the stage for bold decision-making and the management of complex strategic decisions: the sale of a company, building a replacement hospital, competing aggressively in a crowded market, or changing the strategic direction of an organization.

The Financial Imperative

Although there are any number of additional skills and competencies required for an executive role, whether as the president of a university, business entrepreneur, managing partner of a firm, or CEO of a hospital system, none is more vital to personal and corporate success than finance. Every corner office executive interviewed stated in unequivocal terms that "finance is the language of business." Integral to the process of corner office socialization is learning the language of accounting and gaining an understanding of the strategic management of financial resources. Needless to say, these management activities are occurring within the highly volatile, politically charged, and exceedingly complex health care environment, and irrespective of the final outcomes of health care reform and the subsequent rules for the implementation of the Affordable Care Act, executives will need to be equipped with the financial tools to quantify the value their organization provides to consumers and the means to manage their organizations into the future. It is important to bear in mind that as a CEO or principal in a business enterprise, you will be responsible for hiring and supervising the organization's chief financial officer (CFO)—quite a unique and thought-provoking opportunity for a nurse!

As a CEO, you assume fiduciary (a trustee of a corporation who maintains the company's assets in trust) responsibility for your organization. That means that by law, corporate directors and officers hold a trust relationship with the corporation, and they are responsible for overseeing its operations, which includes its financial operations. This trust relationship involves fiduciary duties that corporate directors and officers owe to the corporation, meaning their actions must be in the best interest of the corporation, and they have a duty to avoid conducting business that injures the corporation.

They are responsible for performing their duties in good faith, although some of the myriad technical elements of accounting, analysis, and reporting will be delegated to skilled finance executives. The CEO is charged with making reliable decisions, and under the business judgment rule, when corporate officers and directors perform their duties in good faith and within their authority, they have fulfilled their corporate responsibilities. When officers or directors make a corporate decision, they must rely on accurate information to prevent a breach of their duty of care to the corporation, suggesting that they must be able to rely on accurate financial information in order to make decisions that are in the best interest of the company. The CEO's financial responsibilities include accountability to the governing board, managing the operations of the organization, strategic planning and budgeting, accounting and financial reporting, financial analysis, and the management of investments, including funding strategies.

The governing board or trustees of an enterprise maintain the ultimate responsibility and authority for organizational decisions and, in turn, the financial condition of the organization. The board has the final approval over adoption of the annual budget and is likely to provide, through their finance committee, guidance in setting the budget. It is this governing body that adopts a mission statement that sets the direction for the organization and engages in determining the strategy to achieve that mission and fulfill the commitment to the community served. In a public company, this board represents the interests of the shareholders, whereas in a privately held company, the board often serves in an advisory capacity (Finkler, Jones, & Kovner, 2013).

While the recent Sarbanes-Oxley legislation (see sidebar) on corporate governance requires publicly traded companies to retain the services of independent directors (see nearby note) on their board, privately held firms are not bound by the same rules. Nonetheless, Edward Hess, a distinguished executive in residence and executive director of the Center for Entrepreneurship & Corporate Growth at Emory University's Goizueta Business School, states that in the day-to-day challenge of running a privately owned firm, an independent director with a successful business background can play an invaluable role by offering an outsider's perspective on a company's affairs (Knowledge@ Emory, 2003). Such a person can act as an industry maven when one is called for, a financial expert when internal or external auditing concerns arise, or as an important contact to gain new customers and outside funding sources. More importantly, Hess notes that for private companies transitioning through the various stages in the development of a business, an independent director can help alleviate the growing pains along the way. Independent directors can help in transitioning the entrepreneur and owner of the business from simply being a "doer" to being a manager and ultimately to becoming a leader (Knowledge@ Emory, 2003).

SARBANES-OXLEY ACT

The Sarbanes-Oxley Act of 2002 (Pub.L. 107-204, 116 Stat. 745), also known as the Public Company Accounting Reform and Investor Protection Act and more commonly called Sarbanes-Oxley or SOX, is a U.S. federal law that set new or enhanced standards for all U.S. public company boards, management, and public accounting firms. It is named after sponsors U.S. Senator Paul Sarbanes (D-MD) and U.S. Representative Michael G. Oxley (R-OH). As a result of SOX, top management must now individually certify the accuracy of financial information. In addition, penalties for fraudulent financial activity are much more severe. Also, SOX increased the independence of the outside auditors who review the accuracy of corporate financial statements and increased the oversight role of boards of directors. The bill was enacted as a reaction to a number of major corporate and accounting scandals, including those affecting Enron and Tyco International. These scandals, which cost investors billions of dollars when the share prices of affected companies collapsed, shook public confidence in the nation's securities markets (Wikipedia, n.d.).

NOTE

An independent director is generally defined as a board member without a financial stake in the company or a personal tie to any one of the company's shareholders, founders, management, or staff.

CFOs typically maintain an independent relationship with the board in their role for the organization. The most common areas of CFO interface with the board include membership on the Finance and Audit Committees of the board, routine reporting of financial results, and strategic planning and budgeting.

CEOs are accountable to the board for the financial performance of the organization; therefore, they must be proficient in developing financial policies and monitoring the ongoing performance of the organization to the plan or budget. The board will rely on the CEO's expertise in assessing market trends and service demand and, in collaboration with a multitude of stakeholders including the community and the medical staff, in deciding on the strategic and programmatic direction of the organization. These difficult strategic decisions, which will eventually be approved by the board, include developing new programs to meet community needs or making the tough decision to close a program that may no longer be profitable. The board will look to the CEO to guide the creation of the capital budget, which prioritizes and directs major expenditures toward projects and programs that will maximize the return on the investment and generate profit for the organization.

It is the CEO to whom the board turns for direction and guidance in the execution of their responsibilities. Quorum Health Resources (2011), in its hospital trustee guide, has a suggested checklist for effective financial oversight for boards of directors:

- The board establishes clear and realistic goals for the financial performance of the organization and its assets.

- Financial performance is reviewed regularly using pre-established and measurable operating ratios and other financial indicators.

- The board works with management to create a budget that reflects the board's goals for the organization.

- The board generally understands which services provide a margin for the organization and which lose money and has criteria for determining how much support should be given to those services that lose money.

- The board understands the assumptions used to create the organization's budget and reviews performance compared to the budget regularly.

(Quorum Health Resources, 2011, p. 31)

It is evident that the board must have a trusted relationship with CEOs and experience a great deal of confidence in their financial expertise. It is through the CEO's leadership and oversight that the business succeeds: optimal outcomes, services, or products delivered effectively for a reasonable cost. As a result, the business thrives and grows.

Another strategic responsibility of the CEO and CFO is the management of the financial assets of the organization. Under the watchful guidance of the board, the CEO is responsible for setting the financial funding strategy for the organization—how will the organization fund the operation, raise capital, and grow into the future? All organizations must manage their financial resources, including cash, marketable investments, and accounts receivable. As division directors or product line managers, nurses have learned how to budget and manage financial performance to that plan. They have also gained experience in developing a capital budget and determining the financial return expected on the equipment or program. Managing the financial assets of an organization requires a broader and deeper understanding of economics, investment strategies, funding sources such as bonds or endowments, as well as the importance of managing and collecting cash.

Health care organizations, as a general rule, rely on cash collected from the provision of services as the main source of funding for operations. The intricate web of reimbursement structures (i.e., private insurance, Medicare, and Medicaid) each have a complex set of rules and procedures governing payment, and, especially in an era of economic and political turmoil, managing the receivables is particularly challenging. Many states are bordering on insolvency and, as a result, delaying payments to health care organizations for services they are required to provide. Keeping a complex organization operating in light of dwindling resources is a major challenge and requires strict discipline around vendor contracts and the accounts payable process. Issues with receivables are not isolated to the provider, however. For the nurse entrepreneur or small business owner with a commercial relationship with a health care organization experiencing financial challenges, the organization's accounts receivable concerns quickly become payable issues that have tremendous implications for any vendor or contractor but particularly for small businesses.

The CEO is confronted with the need to manage timely payment of receivables, which is highly dependent on efficient internal systems for correct billing, against the operating necessities and multiple internal and external constituents, often with competing requests. Without sufficient receivables (i.e., cash), the organization is unable to replace aging facilities, keep current with advances in technology, fulfill its responsibility to the community as an employer, and fund the future.

In collaboration with the CFO and board, the corner office executive determines the investment strategy for the organization and manages the banking relationship. How much risk is the organization willing to take? How and where should money be invested to receive the highest return? What banks, investors, or other financial institutions are worthy and ethical partners with a proven record for maximizing the return of investment? Of significant importance is the CEO's role in assuring that the investment strategy is aligned with the mission and values of the organization. This is particularly relevant in a faith-based or even "green"-oriented organization, which may have a preference for investing in funds with a penchant toward social accountability.

The bond rating is exceedingly important to the bottom line of an organization, especially in a volatile marketplace during a depressed economy, when revenues may be less predictable. A bond is a long-term debt instrument under which a borrower agrees to make payments of both interest and principle on particular dates to the holder of the debt (i.e., the bond). In reality, the bondholder is a creditor, because bonds are liabilities to the issuing company. While similar to a term loan, a bond issue is generally registered with the U.S. Securities and Exchange Commission, advertised, offered to the public through investment bankers, and sold to many different investors, sometimes hundreds or thousands of institutional and individual investors.

"Bonds are an advantageous way of obtaining debt for several reasons. First, the borrower obtains the money directly from the ultimate lender and second, bonds tend to disperse risk" (Finkler et al., 2013, p. 331). In contrast to a bank loan, wherein the bank utilizes depositor funds to make loans, with bonds, money is borrowed directly from individuals who might otherwise put their money in a bank. When a bank makes a loan, not only must the depositor make money but the bank itself must make a profit. In the situation of a bond issuance, there is no "middle man" per se, and as a result, the depositor can earn more money off the investment.

The second major advantage is the dispersal of risk. If a bank were to lend an organization $250 million dollars for a capital building project, it would be taking on tremendous risk. If the organization defaulted on the loan, the bank would be faced with substantial losses. In contrast, bonds are divided into many small loans, for example, $5,000 for an individual; therefore, no single person or entity is at risk for the full amount.

While there are several types of bonds typically issued in health care (e.g., corporate, municipal, and mortgage), depending on the corporate structure, ownership model, or intended use of the financing, the priority for the CEO is the overall financial strength of the organization, since the bond rating determines the cost and availability of that money, that is, the interest rate the organization will be required to pay. The primary reason for issuing bonds rather than using conventional debt for a major project, such as a capital building initiative, is the ability to borrow the money at a lower rate of interest. An important determinant of interest rate is risk. If investors perceive an investment to be risky, they will lend the money at a higher rate of interest. A bond rating is assigned by an independent rating agency that evaluates the financial health of an organization as a predictor of its ability to repay the loan. An organization rated AAA, the highest rating available, can borrow money at substantially less interest, because it is more likely that the organization will repay the loan and interest at the prescribed time, therefore making the loan less risky. This is why it is so important that the CEO manage the operation in a financially responsible manner; the ability to meet the needs of the community depends substantially on making astute investments to fund the future.

This is an interesting era as it relates to investment strategy, suggesting that the executive nurse needs to gain a deep understanding of market economics generally and health care economics specifically, coupled with a bit of crystal ball gazing to determine how and where precious dollars should be invested. Many organizations are faced with the need to replace or upgrade their aging physical plant due to changing consumer demands or the implementation of new technology. Yet the health care system of the immediate future would seem to indicate that care will be centered in the community rather than in the acute care hospital, suggesting a very different investment strategy (i.e., urgent care centers, practitioner offices, home health companies). Peter Frost (2012) of *The Chicago Tribune* reported that Chicago area hospitals had spent more than $6.6 billion between April 2009 and April 2011 on new facilities and updates to existing buildings. "The spending spree underscores a race to gain and hold on to market share in one of the most competitive health care markets in the country. It also comes at a time of vast uncertainty in the industry, which faces drastic changes in the way care is delivered and paid for as part of the rollout of the national health care overhaul" (Frost, 2012, p. 1). The nurse CEO and advisors will be obliged to lead the organization through this difficult landscape.

Managing Complexity

The CEO operating in this chaotic environment will be challenged in unprecedented ways because of the shifting landscape: uncertain reform initiatives, unstable financial markets, and workforce challenges. Although money and financial growth are the language of business, these changes will create a more complex environment with different rules of engagement and new partnerships, which will require a distinct management tool set: managing complexity.

In early 2012, Barton, Grant, and Horn interviewed several global business leaders, including the CEOs of DuPont, Deutsche Bank, and Novartis. Although it is often stated that the principles of great leadership are timeless, these leaders of some of the world's largest organizations reported that everything felt different from just a decade earlier. These leaders described that they were operating in a bewildering new environment in which little was certain, the tempo was faster, and the dynamics were increasingly more complex. It certainly sounds as if these leaders were describing health care. Successful CEOs utilize a number of strategies as they struggle to understand the convergence of forces reshaping the business landscape: the pace of innovation, which is increasing exponentially; new technologies; changing workforce demographics; managing complex risk; and volatile financial markets.

In the course of the McKinsey interviews (Barton et al., 2012), Carlos Ghosn of Nissan and Renault discussed the various forms of crises confronted by CEOs, both internal and external, and the different leadership strategies required in each. He contended that internal crises arise from ineffectual management. This might take the form of an insufficient strategy or problems with execution, failure to align stakeholders around the strategy, management of finances and cash flow, or losing sight of market requirements. He contended that business schools prepare senior leaders to effectively deal with these types of crises. External crises, on the other hand, are often difficult to prepare for, since it is not the strategy of the company in question, but rather the company's ability to adapt that strategy to external events. In an era of global market, political, technological, and environmental volatility, with intense feedback loops providing almost real-time reaction to decisions, CEOs are obligated to manage in a disciplined yet imaginative manner.

This new, more public face of leadership often results in the challenge of dealing with constant scrutiny and of acting as the connector in a complex business ecosystem. As the CEO, a leader must be able to address the practical concerns of the job while maintaining and articulating a long-term vision of the purpose of the organization and its role in service to its constituents and the community served—all against the backdrop of transparency and 24/7 media, Twitter, email, and Facebook coverage.

Josef Ackerman of Deutsche Bank told of valuable advice he received early in his CEO career that continues to serve him well: "From now on, you must remember that you are two people. You are the person whom you and your friends know, but you are also a symbol for something. Never confuse the two. Don't take criticism of the symbol (position) as criticism of the person" (Barton et al., 2012).

Contemporary organizations have evolved from creatures that are merely complicated to complex. Complicated systems have a multitude of moving parts, but they typically operate in patterned ways, and as such, it is far easier to predict how a complicated system will behave. While flying an airplane is a technically complicated process, it consists of predictable steps and, as a result, has become astonishingly safe over time. Complex systems, on the other hand, are much more difficult to manage because the outlier is often more significant than the average—the past behavior of a complex system may not predict its future behavior. If you manage a complex organization as if it were simply a complicated organization, serious and costly mistakes may result (Sargut & McGrath, 2011).

By contrast, complicated systems are imbued with features that may operate in patterned ways but whose interactions are constantly changing. Sargut and McGrath (2011) have identified three properties that determine the complexity of an environment. Multiplicity refers to the number of potentially interacting elements. The second, interdependence, relates to how connected those elements are, while the third, diversity, has to do with the degree of heterogeneity within the system. The greater the presence of these three characteristics, the greater the complexity of the system. In contrast to a complicated system in which outcomes can generally be predicted by knowing the starting conditions, in a complex system, the same starting conditions can produce different outcomes depending on the interactions within the system.

The two major issues executives face when managing complexity are (a) the unintended consequences of decisions and (b) difficulty in making sense of a situation; that is, they have a limited view of the situation given their vantage point. By recognizing these limitations, CEOs are able to construct a holistic approach to management that ensures diversity of thought and mitigates the risks often associated with complex decision-making.

Pat O'Donoghue addresses the importance of gaining a wide view of issues and therefore making more grounded decisions through surrounding oneself with individuals with a different skill set than yours: "The ability to develop people is fundamental to any leader's success. For nurses, you first learn how to work with people and motivate them. You gain those skills every day whether interacting with a patient, a doctor, a colleague, or whomever. One of the things that nurses learn early is good communication skills, which are fundamental. You have to listen to what people are trying to tell you, watch their body language, and pay total attention during the interaction. You're not sitting there thinking of your answer before they ask you a question. Another skill nurses master is how to communicate your own ideas. Without mastering these areas, success is not attainable."

Taking a lesson from our clinical experiences, we know that in a complex environment, even the smallest decisions can lead to surprisingly significant results. First is when events interact without anyone meaning for them to. Examples of this abound with surprising magnitude in all aspects of our environment: A change in the timing of a traffic signal causes significant tie-ups miles away; using a chemical to remove unsightly weeds from a garden may impact the wildlife ecosystem in a stream a mile away; a small change in emergency department throughput leads to a significant improvement in patient satisfaction scores.

In the second situation, unintended consequences are based on an aggregate of individual elements rather than a single occurrence. The recent economic "meltdown" was attributable to a multitude of causes—monetary policies keeping interest rates low, the dilution of reasonable credit standards, and the creation of financial instruments that permitted investors to shift risk off their balance sheets, for example—yet no single party from their particular view could see the convergence of all of these forces and the consequences on the entire economic system (Sargut & McGrath, 2011). An example that often plagues CEOs of acute care organizations might be the case in which partnering with a physician practice for the purpose of better integrating services results in a competing group severing ties with the organization and moving business to a competitor across town. While the goal had been a genuine desire to improve services to the community, the outcome for the organization was undermined in the process.

A third scenario occurs when policies and procedures stay in place long after the reasons for their creation have become obsolete. We see this scenario repeated often in health care, whereby a special cause event leads to the creation of an elaborate web of policies or procedures aimed at avoiding the situation in the future. Time may prohibit a thorough study of the circumstances leading up to this event; therefore, the remedy is often overly simplistic and built around today's processes. As the organization and its processes evolve over time, these procedures and rituals add unnecessary complexity and expense, will cease to add value, and will eventually stifle creativity.

The interdependencies within a complex organization cannot be overemphasized, because these connections and interrelationships that are often hidden from the decision-maker. It is important to recognize that CEOs, along with all leaders within an organization, are limited by their vantage point, making it difficult to observe and comprehend the highly diverse array of relationships operating within the enterprise. CEOs are further hampered by cognitive limits to their understanding of the effects of others' actions as well as their own.

Most executives believe that they can absorb and make sense of more information than research suggests. As a result, they may make decisions prematurely and without full comprehension of the consequences for the entire system. We also know that focusing on a single event or activity can prevent us from seeing other priorities (Heywood, Spungin, & Turnbull, 2007; Kerridge, 1997; Sargut & McGrath, 2011). However, the CEO cannot be stymied by lengthy data collection and err on the side of "analysis paralysis." Organizations that are run by committee, where accountability is diffuse and issues are overanalyzed, find themselves at a competitive disadvantage. They are unlikely to take the bold yet thoughtful action required to thrive in this difficult market. In uncertain times, leaders must resist the temptation to cope with complexity by trusting their "gut," since past experience is an unreliable guide to future outcomes. Although these appear to be polar opposite approaches to management, they really suggest that CEOs create a culture of constructive skepticism and surround themselves with highly qualified individuals who are comfortable bringing multiple perspectives to the discussion without fear of challenging the CEO.

Pat Thompson reports that an important element in her management success was working with and through others: "I really had developed, through my various administrative positions, a pretty strong administrative skill set, both with knowledge but also people skills. I guess I have to say that I really believe that to be a dean or a CEO, you obviously have some knowledge, but if you have a strong people skill set, you don't even always have to be a detailed person or have some of these other pieces, if you're smart enough to recognize where your strengths are and what areas you're a little bit weaker in and hire folks in those positions that have the skill set to support what you're trying to do."

Collectively, these problems suggest that complex systems pose challenges in three areas of leadership: forecasting, mitigating risk, and making trade-offs in decision-making. While even the most experienced CEOs experience difficulty in managing complexity, there are several techniques that help them achieve success in the face of overwhelming complexity.

- **See with a microscope and telescope simultaneously.** The CEO must be able to manage the immediacy of the enterprise within a long-term context, in other words, seeing the world in multiple ways at once. A view through the telescope will allow for consideration of opportunities far into the future, always mindful of long-term trends and big dreams, imagining where the organization *could* be 5 or 10 years into the future and then allocating capital and other resources in a way to make it happen. The microscope, on the other hand, affords a critical perspective, encouraging a challenge to conventional wisdom while focusing on the current issues. The talented CEO shifts between the two—far-sightedness and nearsightedness—with ease and speed.

- **Barton et al. (2012) suggest that the CEO needs to compete as a tri-sector athlete.** The environment in which we operate is buffeted by forces from multiple sectors: public, private, and social. Government interventions in health care policy, issues with

unemployment, infrastructure, and environmental concerns are just a few of the global complexities facing
our organizations, requiring nimble and well-informed
leaders at the helm.

- **Stay grounded during a crisis.** As much as we would
  like to leave firefighting to the professional firefighters,
  we spend a great deal of our time doing just that—and
  as complexity grows, so will the portion of CEO time
  devoted to extinguishing the blazes that are ignited
  as a result. Barton et al. (2012) reference a growing
  body of research in psychology, sociology, and neu-
  roscience that highlights the importance of decision
  fatigue. These data imply that attempting to make too
  many decisions at once diminishes the ability to make
  thoughtful decisions at all. Their interviews of CEOs
  from large global firms suggest that prudent CEOs
  reserve crucial decisions for moments when they know
  they will be rested and free from distraction. They also
  noted the importance of sequencing decisions—focusing on key issues first and not after they are depleted
  by lesser matters.

- **Expert CEOs know how to use data to quickly get to
  the problem.** By using context information, we improve our range of decision-making as well as reduce
  the fear surrounding decision-making. We can quickly
  track the response and correct the course. Under
  statistical control, the leader can use experience more
  effectively. These data need to be shared generously
  with managers and employees so that they can be
  enlisted in the creative problem-solving process. There
  is more to data than averages, the only statistic many
  of us remember from our graduate statistics class. By
  averaging data, the nuance of variation is lost, as is the
  identification of those meaningful special causes. The
  CEO is better able to manage complexity by mathematically predicting or forecasting the behavior of a
  system. Sargut and McGrath (2011) state that "in-

stead of extrapolating from irrelevant medians, look to modeling that will give you insight into the system and the ways in which its various elements interact" (p. 73). This will require a deeper understanding of the tools and mathematical modeling widely used in other industries, but the results will produce better, data-driven leadership and financial decision-making.

- **Avoid the tendency to overcontrol.** As we begin to feel the loss of control, it is in our nature to hold on tight and attempt to stop what feels like a free fall. The control loops around many of our organizational processes are meant to direct the system toward the aims leaders have determined. Overcontrolling the system may result in rigidity, which will lengthen response time in problem-solving. The system may never reach a steady state, and instead, the complex interaction of forces can lead to wild oscillations. Well-thought-out delegation when goals have been clearly communicated will minimize conflict and empower staff decision-making while permitting the CEO to stay focused on the strategic priority issues at hand.

- **Heywood et al. (2007) challenge the notion that complexity is necessarily a bad thing,** but rather support a more nuanced perspective that complexity is a challenge to be managed and exploited as a means to generate additional sources of profit and competitive advantage. Managing complexity well can increase the resilience of an enterprise and enhance its ability to adapt to the rapidly changing world. Individual complexity—that is, the way individuals deal with complexity—can be improved by creating detailed operating model choices, clarifying roles, refining key processes, and developing appropriate skills and capabilities among managers and employees. The organization itself can become more complex if managers and employees have the requisite skills to adapt to those changes.

- **Understand in no uncertain terms what drives value in your organization.** When you have minimized the individual complexity—the difficulty employees experience in getting their jobs done—institutional complexity can be exploited to pursue more challenging and value-creating strategies. Companies that are resilient and manage complexity well are simply harder to imitate.

- **Effective organizational design can minimize complexity.** This means eliminating multiple steps in decision-making, eliminating redundancies, creating clear performance targets, and creating clear accountabilities. It also means realigning operating processes with the goal of improving efficiencies at all levels of the organization.

- **Build individual employee and manager capacity through robust education and role development.** This will enable the organization to become "ambidextrous" while increasing the capacity to add value.

- **Avoid reductionist thinking and the inclination to look for a direct cause-and-effect relationship with events.** As humans we have a tendency to look for the single reason to explain an event, and in a simple era this served us well. However, as complexity has become the rule in our organizations, there is rarely a single cause leading to a particular outcome. In fact, it is often the convergence of many systems and individuals trying to do the right thing that produces an outcome. When we see something occur in a complex system, our mind wants to create a narrative to explain what happened, even though cause and effect may be impossible. This inadvertently creates a bias in our thinking with the potential to create a cascade of poor decision-making.

(Barton et al., 2012; Heywood et al., 2007; Kerridge, 1997; Sargut & McGrath, 2011; Sullivan, 2011)

Executive Leadership Lessons

- Seek out a mentor to help hone the basic skills required for the executive suite, particularly finance; look outside of health care for specific expertise.

- Finance is the language of business; therefore, immerse yourself in education around strategic financial management (i.e., the management of investments).

- Develop an understanding of the responsibilities that a CEO or business owner has to the board.

- Learn to understand and manage complexity; be a courageous decision-maker; understand the unintended consequences of decisions; realize that you have a limited view of the situation given your vantage point.

- Learn to seek honest feedback; develop a tough skin whereby you separate feedback on a performance issue or poor decision from you as an individual; quickly study the problem, determine what went wrong, and determine how you might leverage those key learnings as your next opportunity.

- Internal crises arise from ineffectual management. This might take the form of an insufficient strategy or problems with execution, failure to align stakeholders around the strategy, management of finances and cash flow, or losing sight of market requirements.

- External crises, on the other hand, are often difficult to prepare for, since it is not the strategy of the company in question but rather the company's ability to adapt that strategy to external events. In an era of global market, political, technological, and environmental volatility, with intense feedback loops providing almost real-time reaction to decisions, CEOs are obligated to manage in a disciplined yet imaginative manner.

- As the CEO, a leader must be able to address the practical concerns of the job while maintaining and articulating a long-term vision of the purpose of the organization and its role in service to its constituents and the community served.

- When managing complexity, remember (a) the unintended consequences of decisions and (b) the difficulty in making sense of a situation, because you will have a limited view of the situation given your vantage point. By recognizing these limitations, you will be able to construct a holistic approach to management that ensures diversity of thought and mitigates the risks often associated with complex decision-making.

- Successful CEOs create a culture of constructive skepticism and surround themselves with highly qualified individuals who are comfortable bringing multiple perspectives to the discussion without fear of challenging the CEO.

- See with a microscope and telescope simultaneously; you must be able to manage the immediacy of the enterprise within a long-term context, in other words, seeing the world in multiple ways at once.

- Stay grounded during a crisis. As much as we would like to leave firefighting to the professional firefighters, we spend a great deal of our time doing just that—and as complexity grows, so will the portion of CEO time devoted to extinguishing the blazes that are ignited as a result.

- Avoid the tendency to overcontrol. As we begin to feel the loss of control, it is in our nature to hold on tight and attempt to stop what feels like a free fall.

- Expert CEOs know how to use data to quickly get to the problem. By using context information, we improve our range of decision-making as well as reduce the fear surrounding decision-making.

- Challenge the notion that complexity is necessarily a bad thing, but rather support a more nuanced perspective that complexity is a challenge to be managed and exploited as a means to generate additional sources of profit and competitive advantage.

References

Barton, D., Grant, A., & Horn, M. (2012). Leading in the 21st century. *McKinsey Quarterly, 3*, 30-47.

Chreim, S., Williams, B. E., & Hinings, C. R. (2007). Interlevel influences on the reconstruction of professional role identity. *Academy of Management Journal, 50*(6), 1515-1539.

Finkler, S. A., Jones, C. B., & Kovner, C. T. (2013). *Financial management for nurse managers and executives* (4th ed.). St. Louis, MO: Elsevier.

Frost, P. (2012, February 19). Chicago area sees hospital building boom. *The Chicago Tribune.* Retrieved from http://articles. chicagotribune.com/2012-02-19/business/ct-biz-0219-hospital-expansion-20120219_1_million-new-hospital-hospital-building-boom-edward-hospital

Gibson, D. E. (2003). Developing the professional self-concept: Role model construals in early, middle, and late career stages. *Organization Science, 14*(5), 591-610.

Healthcare Leadership Alliance and the American College of Healthcare Executives. (2011). *ACHE Healthcare Executive Competencies Assessment Tool.*

Heywood, S., Spungin, J., & Turnbull, D. (2007). Cracking the complexity code. *McKinsey Quarterly, 2*, 84-95.

Kerridge, D. (1997). Managing complexity. *Journal for Quality & Participation, 20*, 60.

Knowledge@Emory. (2003). How should privately owned firms structure the board of directors? Retrieved from http:// knowledge.emory.edu/article.cfm?articleid=701

Quorum Health Resources. (2011). *Hospital trustee quick reference guide*. Brentwood, CA: QHR Learning Institute.

Sarbanes-Oxley Act. (n.d.). In *Wikipedia*. Retrieved January 23, 2013, from http://en.wikipedia.org/wiki/Sarbanes–Oxley_Act

Sargut, G., & McGrath, R. G. (2011). Learning to live with complexity. *Harvard Business Review, 89*(9), 68-76.

Sullivan, T. (2011). Embracing complexity. *Harvard Business Review, 89*(9), 88-92.

Chapter 5
The Rules of Engagement: The Buck Stops Here— The Board

"When I had a General Assistance Medical Program, we used to do a satisfaction survey. When I would get a good one, I would send it down to the county board supervisor of that area and just say, 'I know you have many priorities, but I just wanted you to see how your decisions are affecting this patient's life.' That was a way to keep the face of the program in front of them so that they understood these are real people at the other end. These are real people with real needs. These aren't just numbers. You have to do a lot of advocating in a type of position like mine."

–Paula Lucey, September 2012

"I learned about board management through doing it and through watching what made other people effective when they worked with boards," says Ann Scott Blouin. Each board is different, she says. "The board was very different at Northwestern than at McNeal and certainly than at Ernst & Young. What makes the board tick, the culture of the board, the structure of the board, the board committees—all are unique to each organization.

"Board management skills are really important; the board is not the same thing as the leadership inside the organization." Unfortunately, she says, "the goal of the board and working effectively with the board is something that is not typically taught in nursing school or graduate school."

✳ The role of the board is governance. Governance is the act of governing and relates to decisions that define expectations, grant power, and verify performance. For-profit boards and nonprofit boards are the two major board classifications. For-profit boards are usually associated with corporations and are owned by their stockholders. Their chief purpose is to increase stockholder wealth. For-profit boards are usually small, and their board members are paid. Nonprofit boards are usually owned by the community and exist to serve a community need. These boards are usually large and made up of unpaid volunteers. By and large, hospital boards are nonprofit boards (although there are some for-profit hospitals). Table 5.1 shows some clear distinctions between for-profit and nonprofit organizations.

TABLE 5.1 Distinctions Between For-Profit and Nonprofit Organizations

FOR-PROFIT CORPORATIONS	NONPROFIT CORPORATIONS
Owned by stockholders	Owned by the public
Generate money for the owners	Serve the public
Success is making sizeable profit	Success is meeting needs of the public
Board members are usually paid	Board members are usually unpaid volunteers

FOR-PROFIT CORPORATIONS	NONPROFIT CORPORATIONS
Members can make very sizeable incomes	Members should make reasonable, not excessive, incomes
Money earned over and above that needed to pay expenses is kept as profit and distributed to owners	Money earned over and above that needed to pay expenses is retained as surplus and should be spent soon on meeting the public need (the nonprofit can earn profit from activities not directly related to the nonprofit's mission; however, the nonprofit often has to pay taxes over a certain amount)
CEO is often on the board of directors, and sometimes is the president of the board	Conventional wisdom suggests that the CEO (often called the "executive director") not be on the board
Usually not exempt from paying federal, state/provincial, and local taxes	Can often be exempt from federal taxes, and some state/provincial and local taxes, if the nonprofit was granted tax-exempt status from the appropriate governmental agency
Money invested in the for-profit usually cannot be deducted from the investor's personal tax liability	Money donated to the nonprofit can be deducted from the donor's personal tax liability if the nonprofit was granted charitable status from the appropriate government agency

Adapted from McNamara (2008)

Nurse leaders can bring a wealth of knowledge and perspective to the board table about the daily experience of providing health care to patients. They also have insight into the needs and concerns of other hospital stakeholders, such as employees and physicians, as they work together with them to provide care and service that is effective, efficient, safe, and high in quality.

However, being on a health care organization board requires the ability to see the bigger picture as well and to grapple with and address fundamental issues of organizational identity, beliefs, and purpose. These are the issues that boards focus on when they discharge their responsibilities for developing the organization's mission, vision, and values and setting strategy to achieve them on behalf of the key stakeholders the organization serves.

Unlike for-profit organizations, whose primary obligation is to increase the wealth of their shareholders, nonprofit hospitals typically serve a variety of stakeholders. Patients, physicians, employees, the broader community, and legislative and regulatory bodies are examples of hospital stakeholders—those individuals or groups who are greatly influenced by the hospital and have a vested interest in its success.

While for-profit companies are clearly focused on maximizing returns to their shareholders, the needs and concerns of nonprofit organization stakeholders are often more diverse and may even conflict with each other. When asked what they most need from a hospital, patients might place high-quality care at the top of the list. Legislators and regulators, on the other hand, may focus first on making care more cost effective. That is why it is important for health care organizations and their boards to understand who their primary stakeholders are and to identify what they most want and need from the organization.

Nurses on Boards

Research on nonprofit hospital governing boards indicates that only about 2% of their members are nurses. We believe that needs to change. Considering the pivotal role that nurses play in the health care industry, their experience, and their direct and significant interactions with patients, who better to serve in these roles?

The value nurses can bring to the board table has been acknowledged and supported by many health care leaders. Donald M. Berwick, MD, president and CEO of the Institute for Health Care Improvement, noted, "It is key that nurses be as involved as physicians, and I think boards should understand that the performance of the organization depends as much on the well-being, engagement, and capabilities of nursing and nursing leaders as it does on physicians. I would encourage a much closer relationship between nursing and the board" (Berwick, 2005, p. 7).

In 2007, the Center for Healthcare Governance's Blue Ribbon Panel on Health Care Governance recommended that boards "include physicians, nurses and other clinicians on the board. Their clinical competence and viewpoints are valuable to other board members and will help the board better understand the needs and concerns of several of the organization's stakeholders" (Center for Healthcare Governance, 2007).

A 2009 Grant Thornton LLP study of governance in community health systems urged that "[a]ll boards should consider enriching their membership with greater racial and gender diversity; they also should consider the appointment of highly respected and experienced nursing leaders as voting members of the board to complement physician members and strengthen clinical input in board deliberations" (Prybil et al., 2009, p. 44). The study also said, "Engaging leaders in the nursing profession on hospital and health system boards has not yet become the norm, nor has it been accepted as a benchmark of good governance. However, given the importance of nursing in the provision of patient care, it seems likely that the idea of engaging nurses on boards and board committees will receive growing consideration in the future" (p. 12).

What do nurses bring to the table?

- Credibility with policymakers, employees, health plan administrators, physicians, and executives

- Public trust—nursing is a top-ranked profession

- The ability to identify and triage problems

- An understanding of issues concerning hospital staff and effective approaches to employee retention

- Awareness of community health needs

Board service brings valuable benefits and awesome responsibility. Connie, who has extensive board experience, both within and outside of health care and the not-for-profit environment, is a strong proponent of board service and the recruitment of nurses to serve on health care boards. Through her role as CEO of Best on Board, an organization that provides online and in-person training, and board certification for health care board members, she provides current and prospective members with the knowledge and information they need to succeed in these roles.

Nurses can benefit in many ways through board service. Board service allows trustees to:

- Set policy that guides care delivery

- Influence resource allocation decisions in ways that maximize stakeholder benefit

- Set strategy to help ensure the future health of a vital community resource

- Assume a valued community leadership role

The hospitals that nurses serve clearly benefit as well. Health care boards and hospital CEOs can take steps to increase the numbers of nurses in governance roles. They can:

- Seek nurse leaders from within and outside of their organizations to serve on the board. Schools of nursing and other community organizations, such as the American Cancer Society, American Heart Association, or Visiting Nurses Association, are good resources to tap.

- Support and encourage nurse leaders within their organizations to prepare for board service by educating themselves on health care governance issues and board roles and responsibilities.

- Work with organizations, such as the Robert Wood Johnson Foundation, that have developed initiatives to help nurses become hospital board members.

What can nurses do to position themselves for such roles? Understanding the health care governance landscape is an important first step for nurses to take on the path to pursuing board service. Governance reform activities in the for-profit and nonprofit sectors over the past decade are demanding increased performance and accountability for governing boards. The American Hospital Association's blue ribbon panels on health care governance and development of trustee core competencies and an expert panel convened by BoardSource to determine principles that empower exceptional governance are examples of efforts that provide guidance to help boards respond to these demands.

It is important that nurses consider securing membership on a nonprofit board. Because boards require a person's time, talent, and intellectual treasures, it is important to determine which board is best for you to pursue. ✳

Assessing Your Potential Board

As you begin to consider how you might contribute to organizations through membership on various boards, it is important to approach this task strategically. The value you attain from board participation can be greatly enhanced through both the contacts you will make and the things you will learn about effective governance.

So your first step will be identifying the boards on which you are interested in participating. Then, consider the following:

1. Why are you attracted to this organization?

2. What are the key problems and accomplishments of the board?

3. Who are the existing board members and what are their skill sets?

4. Are you willing to devote 4 to 6 hours/month to this board?

5. Are you willing to give or get money for the organization?

6. What skills and expertise do you have to assist this board and organization?

Once you have identified a board that you are interested in joining, it is necessary to gain access to that board. It is essential that you create a résumé that reflects the expertise you bring to the board. You may know one of the existing board members, and that will provide you an approach to the organization. You may want to volunteer for the organization to obtain some experience. Giving and getting money for the organization always capture the board's attention and can provide access to the board.

Your Role in Corporate Governance

Eighteen percent of America's gross domestic product goes to health care; that suggests there are hundreds of for-profit organizations that sell products and services related to health care. For-profit companies often want board members who have business experience, financial acumen, and governance experience. In addition, nurses—because of their immersion in the clinical issues that impact health care organizations—often have health care knowledge that is very valuable to these health care-related companies. With the Institute of Medicine's (IOM's) call for more involvement of nurses on boards through *The Future of Nursing: Leading Change, Advancing Health* (IOM, 2010), the value that nurses can bring has never been more on the radar screen of many of these organizations.

Your participation on a board is serious business. For-profit boards are overseen by the Securities and Exchange Commission (SEC). Corporate boards, and their members, are accountable to understand and operate within the SEC rules and regulations.

Service on a nonprofit board is an excellent way to secure the governance experience that will prepare you for a position on a for-profit board.

Participation on a nonprofit board is an easier first step than attempting to break into the for-profit world of governance. In many cases, networking with local nonprofit directors and expressing your interest in serving can help you to land a spot on a board. Once you've gained experience here and have a good idea of what is required of board members and how you can contribute most effectively based on the expertise and knowledge you bring, you may want to consider participation on a for-profit board.

For-profit boards usually use executive search firms to identify potential board members. Nurse leaders can submit their résumés to these search firms for consideration to serve on corporate boards. In doing so, think back to the questions formerly presented and gear your résumé to the specific board you are approaching. Given your knowledge of the make-up of the board, the potential gaps in knowledge and experience that may exist, and how your core competencies could help to fill those gaps, position yourself through your résumé in a way that clearly establishes the value you might bring to the board. Again, a key value that nurses can bring to boards is their health care experience and direct and extensive contact with patients.

Because nurses are relatively new to board experience, and because many boards today, particularly in the for-profit world, are still populated primarily by males, breaking into this predominantly male network and navigating the inevitably political nature of these experiences can be challenging.

In many environments, gender issues need to be carefully navigated. Noted Therese, "Working in organizations where I was finding myself the first woman stepping into a position, I learned that, number one, it's up to you. You need to own a great piece of how you're going to be accepted into those fairly elite ranks.

"It is incumbent upon you to develop the analytical skills, to read the political situation that you're walking into and—without compromising your own values, your own perspectives, or your own authenticity—to figure out how to work in the political situations in which you find yourself. By doing that, incredible doors open for us as nurses and as women."

Working With Your Company's Board

In addition to gaining experience through serving on boards, nurses can also learn about boards and how they work through their own organization's board. Nurse leaders frequently work with board members. Most hospital nurse executives attend board meetings and work with the board in the areas of strategic planning, quality of care, and patient satisfaction, among others.

It is essential that nurse executives seek opportunities to present to the board, to staff board committees, and to educate the board about patient care issues and opportunities. Nurse leaders should also ensure that their organization has nurses as board members. Because the board determines the CEO's succession plan and appoints the CEO, nurse leaders who aspire to the corner office should ensure that they are considered for promotion within the organization.

Creating Your Company's Board

For entrepreneurial nurses who have started their own companies, establishing a board of directors—even when not required by your organizational structure—can bring value to your organization. A board can bring expert skills and experience to assist nurse leaders and their leadership team. When Connie was building CurranCare, she created a board of advisors. The CurranCare board was composed of national leaders in health care, a corporate finance expert, and an expert in corporate mergers and acquisitions. Small companies cannot afford to hire, and usually do not require, this type of full-time assistance. Board appointments can provide easy access to this expertise. To secure this type of talent, it is essential to give your advisors or board members equity in the company as well as payment for their services. Although some entrepreneurs are hesitant to give away equity, it is essential to realize that great talent will help grow the equity and increase everyone's investment.

At CurranCare, the board met quarterly and reviewed the company's performance, planning, and company development. A "big four" auditing firm was employed to provide audited financials at each board meeting. Connie wanted to simulate the functioning of a public company to prepare for acquisition by a larger organization at some future time.

Whether in a nonprofit, for-profit, or entrepreneurial environment, a board of directors brings significant value to the organization. Regardless of your role, make sure that you are capitalizing on experiences at the board level to deepen your expertise and the ability to contribute to organizations' missions as they serve their constituents.

There has never been a better time for nurses to step up and take on the responsibilities and opportunities of board leadership. As Pat O'Donoghue says, "Nursing today is making an extraordinary contribution to the well-being of our society and to health care. I feel that we're standing as we should to achieve our potential to make a difference, the potential for change, the potential for making people's lives better, and the potential to build a stronger health care system. Clearly, it is in the hands of the nursing profession more than it's ever been before."

Executive Leadership Lessons

- In both for-profit and nonprofit boards, planning, budgeting, and performance measurement systems are essential.

- Both types of boards add value to society in different ways.

- Both types of organizations can grow, transform, merge, or die.

- Good governance is essential for the success of all organizations.

- Nurse leaders possess the knowledge, skills, and values to be excellent board members.

- The Institute of Medicine has identified the need for nurses to play a greater role in the governance of health care organizations.

References

Berwick, D. (2005). Great boards ask tough questions: What to expect from management on quality. *Boardroom Press, 16*, 2-7.

Center for Healthcare Governance. (2007). *2007 Blue Ribbon Panel report: Building an exceptional board: Effective practices for health care governance.* Chicago, IL: Author.

Institute of Medicine (IOM). (2010). *The future of nursing: Leading change, advancing health.* Washington, DC: The National Academics Press.

McNamara, C. (2008). *Field guide to developing, operating and restoring your nonprofit board.* Minneapolis, MN: Authenticity Consulting, LLC.

Prybil, L., Levey, S., Peterson, R., Heinrich, D., Brezinski, P., Zamba, G., . . . Roach, W. (2009). *Governance in high-performing community health systems.* Chicago, IL: Grant Thornton LLP.

Chapter 6
Reinventing Your Personal Brand

"Whether for-profit or not-for-profit, the biggest crime a company can commit is the failure to make a profit, because then you're a weak company with weak opportunities, whether you're not-for-profit or profit. You have to be able to have a strong infrastructure and reinvestment strategy."

–P. K. Scheerle, September 2012

Self-development is an ongoing process and an important factor in your success. Whether the corner office you wish to land in is in a hospital, a university, or a business of your own, there are a number of skills that you need to hone to ensure that both the journey and the destination will be as fruitful as possible.

When Connie decided to be a nurse, it was not with the idea that she would ultimately pursue an EdD, or that she would become a serial entrepreneur. In fact, she says when she initially began her career, she did not really even have an interest in leadership. "I just had an enormous interest in trying to learn as much as I could to be a safe, confident nurse and not to hurt anybody," she says. But, once she had that mastered, she began seeing opportunities where she felt she might make a difference. "I started looking around a little bit and thinking, 'I could do this better, or at least as good as, the people I saw doing it," she says.

What draws most of us into the nursing profession, initially, of course, is our strong desire to help others—to care for others. Few embark on this journey with the thought, "Someday I want to sit in the corner office." That is a passion that develops over time. As Pat Thompson tells us, "It's probably something you hear from a lot of people of my generation, but it was just the idea of helping people and wanting to make a difference" that drew her to nursing.

But what leads those in the nursing profession to the top? What are the traits and characteristics that set them apart?

Barrick and Mount (1991) focused in their study on the traits of extroversion, emotional stability, agreeableness, conscientiousness, and openness to experience in relation to job proficiency, training proficiency, and personnel data. Although all factors were important for certain types of positions or in certain situations, the one factor that showed up most consistently as correlated with success was conscientiousness—being careful, thorough, responsible, organized, and planful—certainly skills that are common among nurses.

Another study (Judge, Cable, Boudreau, & Bretz, 1995), found that the characteristics we often perceive as defining our success are not the same as the variables that lead to *objective* career success. Results obtained from a sample of 1,388 U.S. executives suggested that demographic, human capital, motivational, and organizational variables explained significant variance in objective career success and career satisfaction. Most notable, the findings suggested that educational level, quality, prestige, and degree type all predicted financial success.

Consider the increasing number of nurses who are going on to complete advanced degrees, considering their registered nurse degree a step along the way to further education. Certainly the nurses we have talked to did just that and, without exception, they believe that their pursuit of these credentials was instrumental in leading them to their current roles.

What Does It Take to Get to the Top?

When they consider the skills that best positioned them for a seat in the corner office, the nurses we interviewed pointed to a number of important traits and characteristics. But underpinning all of these traits was the need for flexibility and balance—being flexible to address the myriad opportunities and challenges that will come your way and finding a way to balance competing demands of personal and professional priorities.

Life experiences can help shape our level of comfort with change and lead to a flexible outlook on life and all that it may put in our paths. Pat Thompson's father was a fighter pilot in the Air Force, so she moved frequently as a child. The longest length of stay in one place, she says, was about 4 years; the shortest about 3 months. "Some of my strengths and skill sets around flexibility and around working with diverse people and populations developed because I grew up in the military," she says.

Balance is important for all of us—juggling the many demands of our personal and professional lives and the needs of those who depend on us, whoever they may be. The myth of "having it all" is increasingly being challenged.

For the most part, says Therese, she was able to find the balance that she needed for both a successful personal life and a successful career. Being up-front about her needs and expectations, and being willing to let others help, were important to help her achieve this balance. "I found that by letting my colleagues know what was important to me—that I was a mom and that I had a young family and that there were some things that I needed to make priorities—was very important. I was always very, very up-front about this. And I always found that my administrative colleagues understood that, and respected it, and I was able to help them be able to stay engaged with their families as well.

"I remember on a number of occasions saying to my hospital president, 'Let me take that late night meeting, because I know your son has a soccer game. Why don't you let me do that?' We were able to work that out to everyone's benefit so that no one's family felt neglected in that process."

Everybody must find the balance that is right for them, notes Rhonda Anderson, who believes that she, her husband, and their children were able to find a balance that worked well for them. "We had a belief, and I definitely had this belief, that children are only the age they are once—they're 2 once, or 5 once—so it's very important for us to have the experiences with them. We never missed an experience."

Paula Lucey acknowledges that she, like others, has had to deal with her own struggles about taking care of self and having some balance. It is important, she says, "to really pay attention to your own health and your own mental health. Some days I'd be good at that, and other days I'd be not so good at that. But I think it's a really important skill to have."

Women are not the only ones who struggle with finding work/life balance, notes P. K. Scheerle. "Male or female, mother or father, if you are going to be a CEO of a meaningful organization, you are going to give something up. To think that anyone has it all all the time is a lie and foolish," she says. "But it's no more so for a female executive who's a mother than it is for a male executive who's a father. Every CEO gives up the same things. Whether you're married or unmarried, whether you have children or you don't, you must still juggle to make your life work; it's really no different. There are times when I am all in for my family, for whatever reason, planned or unplanned. And, there are times when I am all in for my business, planned or unplanned."

The word *balance,* though, suggests Connie, may lead to unrealistic expectations. "Work/life balance is a nice thing to think about, but in reality, life is kind of like a Slinky. We're moving through time and space and sometimes things seem very balanced and moving along just right, and then the next day, you're coming around the bend and there's a big challenge in front of you."

The balance—if there really is true balance—is more of a mental construct, she suggests. "You have to sort of be able to work it out in your head, I think. It's important if you can have people who support you, but I really think it's a mental construct to feel like you're balanced."

Pat O'Donoghue has a similar perspective: "You can do your very best and give as much as you can, but I have learned that you can only give what you have to offer at any point in time," she says. Along the way, she says, "you learn many skills as you try to manage home and work. You get very good at prioritizing, compartmentalizing; you get especially good at time management. You adapt." Nurses, she says, are generally good adapters. "We adapt to whatever is coming our way on any given day," she says. "You do what you have to do. But you never lose sight of what the endpoint is. You do the best that you can; that's all that anybody can ask of you."

As we work to find balance, we are also working to overcome our weaknesses and build upon our strengths. Self-development is an important part of career progression. Those who do it well progress; those who do not may find themselves languishing in a role that is neither personally nor professionally stimulating. The good news, according to the experts, is that we can gain more by focusing on our strengths than by perseverating over our weaknesses.

Self-Development: Working on Your Rough Edges and Polishing Your Jewels

The ability to accurately identify both the rough edges that may be holding you back and the hidden jewels that may be just waiting to be revealed can be challenging. After all, each of us is our own worst critic. Sometimes we do not see clearly what others clearly see. Other times we are overly critical of traits that others either do not view as downfalls or may not even notice.

It is important to note, though, that failure is not always bad. In fact, many of us have learned the most from our failures. Thomas Watson, Sr., who led IBM, is reported to have said, "The fastest way to succeed is to double your failure rate" (Farson & Keyes, 2002, p. 64). That is certainly true for innovative companies that try and fail frequently until they discover the next best thing. It is also true for nurses as we navigate through an increasingly complex and constantly changing health care environment.

But people are afraid to fail. If you are one of those people, that is another important area for you to work on in terms of your own self-development. In addition, your tolerance—or intolerance—of failure will also impact how effectively you lead others.

Farson and Keyes (2002) provide some insights into the traits and characteristics of what they call "failure tolerant leaders." Through their research with business, political, sports, and science leaders, Farson and Keyes point to a number of characteristics common to failure-tolerant leaders:

- They break down the social and bureaucratic barriers that separate them from their followers.

- They engage at a personal level with those they lead.

- They openly admit their own mistakes instead of trying to cover them up or shift blame.

- They try to eliminate destructive competitiveness.

- They push people to see beyond the traditional definitions of success and failure.

(Farson & Keyes, 2002)

Marcus Buckingham and Donald O. Clifton (2001), authors of *First, Break All the Rules* and *Now, Discover Your Strengths,* publications that were based on extensive Gallup research, are strong proponents of doing exactly what the second title suggests—discovering (and focusing on) strengths. This is counterintuitive for those of us who have been trained through our childhoods and well into our careers to work hard to overcome our weaknesses. Gallup research suggests, however, that we are better served by identifying those things that we do well and focusing on ways we can do them better. A corollary to this for leaders, of course, is to surround themselves with others whose strengths balance their own weaknesses.

By the time we begin to consider a corner office opportunity, it is presumed that we are well immersed in a successful career; we have experienced our share of successes, demonstrated our capabilities in creative ways, grown businesses under another's direction, or even reached a pinnacle in academic preparation. We have demonstrated that we can be counted on to do the right thing at the right time for all the right reasons; in other words, we have become the "go-to" nurse leader because we deliver. While these herculean talents have gotten us to where we are today, they may not be enough to get us where we would like to be. "What got you here won't get you there," as Connie likes to say. Remember what Henry Wadsworth Longfellow famously stated: "We judge ourselves by what we feel capable of doing, while others judge us by what we have already done." (n.d.).

This may be particularly challenging for nurses who, by virtue of our education, clinical careers, and typical professional progression, are often characterized as clinical leaders of nursing departments or managers of product lines, again with a primary clinical emphasis. But just as a product may be rebranded or an industry reinvented, we have an opportunity to rebrand ourselves as a means of being seen as leaders with the breadth and depth of experience and the capability to accomplish astounding feats in the corner office.

The Process of Rebranding

Dorie Clark (2011), a consultant who helps organizations build their brands, has applied some of the same strategies to brand redo's for individuals. She contends that people reinvent themselves all the time—to take on a new challenge, shift into more meaningful work, or even as a means to alter perceptions that have hindered career progress. Taking responsibility for your personal brand may signal the difference between continuing in your current role or catapulting yourself into a corner office trajectory.

 She suggests a four-step process to a personal brand reboot.

The First Step

The first step is to clearly define your destination. As in planning for any journey, you need to have a very clear vision of where you intend to end up. Some might even suggest that describing your eventual endpoint, whether CEO, business owner, or college president, is the first step in manifesting that outcome. Being crystal clear with your goals will not only attract individuals into your professional sphere with the ability to add value to your plan by providing coaching or network support, but you also will see opportunities present themselves in new and interesting ways. The offer to work on a project in another area of the enterprise might provide the opening you have been looking for to round out your résumé and become more familiar with a wider view of the operation. Or an offer to manage departments outside of nursing may provide introductions to individuals with the political capital to facilitate your journey. Remember, what got you here will not get you there; therefore, you will need new contacts and additional experiences to get you where you want to go.

Rebranding is impossible without first determining how and where to invest your energy. It is only after you create this image that you can begin to construct a plan for the journey. If you are looking to stay within your current organization, there are formal programs available to learn additional skills, for example, financial management, strategic planning, investment strategy, or corporate governance. There are online, virtual, or residency-based educational and certificate programs available for this self-development. Several examples are noted here, but there are also a number of programs and classes available at colleges and universities in your geographic area. Many also offer online options as well:

- The Robert Wood Johnson Fellows program: http://rwjf.org/content/rwjf/en/research-publications/find-rwjf-research/2011/05/robert-wood-johnson-foundation-executive-nurse-fellows.html

- University of Pennsylvania's Wharton School of Business executive program: http://executiveeducation.wharton.upenn.edu/open-enrollment/health-care-programs/Fellows-Program-Management-Nurse-Executives.cfm?searchPos=1

- Harvard Business School's executive leadership programs: http://www.exed.hbs.edu/landing/Pages/clpcomparison.aspx?utm_campaign=US+-+Brand+-+Executive+Education&utm_medium=ppc&utm_source=google&utm_term=harvard_executive_programs&gclid=CI2wu4rxirMCFUZgMgod62kAqg

- Keller Graduate School of Management business certificate programs: http://get-started.keller.edu/keller-micrositev2-gradcertificate/grad-certificates-366Z-1289F5.html

- The University of Chicago Booth School of Business executive programs: http://booth.chicagoexec.net/home/home.aspx

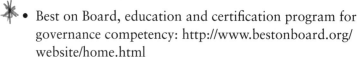

- Best on Board, education and certification program for governance competency: http://www.bestonboard.org/website/home.html

- Sigma Theta Tau International: http://www.nursingsociety.org

In addition to adding to your management repertoire through formal educational programs, it is important to inform your current CEO of your career aspirations and ask for the opportunity to work on projects or attend meetings that will provide exposure to a wider perspective of the enterprise and present greater opportunities for introductions to key individuals both within and outside of the organization. For example, attendance at board meetings will provide exposure to key community leaders as well as provide a viewpoint on the board's fiduciary responsibility for the organization and the data they need to fulfill that critical role.

The board's role is different from management's in that the board generally decides why the organization exists, who the customers are, and what services should be provided. The board also is responsible for assuring the quality and cost of those services, as well as who will lead the organization in the role of CEO. The board clearly cannot do its job effectively without a talented management team to lead operations and provide the information the board requires to function effectually. Management's role includes the development and execution of the plan on how to reach customers, how to best optimize the services determined by the board, how to run operations efficiently and effectively, how to operationalize the board's goals, and whom to hire to make this all happen (Quorum Health Resources, 2011).

Therese had a conversation with a chief nurse colleague not long ago. Her colleague was lamenting that a vice president was promoted into the president role at one of the system's many hospitals. She felt that there were several chief nursing officers (CNOs) within the system equally qualified to step into the corner office and wondered why they were not chosen. When Theresa asked her colleague if the CNOs had made their desire to be included in the succession plan known to corporate leaders, the reply was no—they assumed they would be tapped for promotion based on performance in their current role. This example illustrates the mistaken belief that opportunities will present themselves without deliberate planning; careers are too important to be left to serendipity. By announcing career goals, you will be able to avail yourself of opportunities for development that will position you for the next corner office position.

The Second Step

The second step in your personal rebranding is learning to leverage your points of difference: how you might think about leveraging your skills and experience as a nurse as a key differentiator in your quest for the corner office. This is an opportunity to think long and hard about your unique selling proposition, that is, the part of you that people will remember, your unique value-add. Is there an opportunity to talk about the fact that you added an entire repertoire of financial skills on top of your clinical leadership experience, making you uniquely qualified to lead an acute care organization? Or might you be able to leverage the fact that you developed the clinical technology strategic plan, led the proposal evaluation process for a new vendor, or directed the implementation of a hospital information system in your quest to become the CEO of a consulting firm focused on clinical technology?

Therese was able to leverage her experience as a CNO with responsibility for budgeting and deploying hundreds of nurses in the pursuit for venture capital to begin a business focused on mathematically right-sizing the clinical workforce. The fact that she had walked the walk and could speak from firsthand experience about the challenges in deploying staff gave her a decided edge. The venture capital investors found this intellectual capital very compelling, and rather than evaluating an abstract concept, they were able to understand the challenges the CNO faced in budgeting and deploying staff and how this solution would benefit them.

The Third Step

The third step in your personal rebranding is to develop a narrative around your key differentiators. Clark (2011) refers to this step as developing a coherent narrative that explains exactly (and confidently) how your past fits into your present. Arguably, this is an easier task when one is moving sequentially up the organizational chart; managers of departments can more easily demonstrate their capability to assume more strategic responsibility by pointing to operational outcomes that suggest they are ready to take on a larger span of control. This narrative, while more challenging to develop when jumping into a corner office trajectory, is easier than you might think.

Clark (2011) suggests, just as when rebranding a product, to not forget about your past but rather to create a narrative consistent with that experience. "In my former (or current) role, I . . ." and "I think that the big picture perspective I gained has uniquely positioned me to . . . ." The goal is to turn a potential weakness (i.e., lack of governance experience) into a substantial strength: "I have a unique view of the impact of our services on our customer." An important caveat is to *never* explain your transition in terms of your personal interests: "I am on a journey to find the role I am best suited for." While your passion should drive this journey, the corner office is not the location for conducting self-discovery, although much soul searching is required prior to the start of the journey.

The Fourth Step

Once the narrative has been constructed, you will need to reintroduce yourself to your existing network. As unbelievable as it may seem, most of your colleagues outside of your immediate network are not watching your career with rapt interest. This means that their recollection of you and your accomplishments is several years out of date, and this phenomenon can be leveraged to your best interest. It presents an opportunity to engage your network using the new narrative and strategically reeducate them on the rebranded you.

As you think about creating your narrative, it is important to consider those differentiating characteristics that will elevate your candidacy for the corner office position. It is important to keep in mind that the environment in which the corner office resides is exponentially more complex and chaotic than even a few years ago. It has been said that the effective CEO must have the skill to see around corners. Two critical leadership characteristics demonstrated by highly sought-after CEOs are adaptability and the ability to regain one's footing after adversity.

Developing Adaptability and Resilience

An extraordinary characteristic exhibited by all of the corner office executives is their remarkable resilience in the face of professional adversity. In fact, many of them were hard pressed to identify a career failure or disappointment, because they had leveraged that misstep into their next success. They did not get stuck in "what if" or "why me" but rather quickly assessed the situation, identified what they could have done to produce a better outcome, then quickly used that opportunity as a springboard to the next success.

The contemporary organization exists against the backdrop of an increasingly complex environment, and as a result, a CEO must balance the agility required to thrive amidst the chaos with the need to create a culture where employees and other stakeholders are secure and confident and able to successfully execute the goals of the organization. Recovering from adversity is a requisite skill of the corner office executive.

How do you react to adversity? What is your instinctual response when things do not go well, and control seems out of reach for the moment? Is your go-to reaction anger or rigid overcontrol, or do you turn your disappointment inward as dejection or victimization? Or do you deny the worst and operate as if it were business as usual? Actually, as nurses we have had the opportunity to develop the aptitude to deal with adversity in our clinical roles. We drill and simulate worst case scenarios relentlessly—cardiac arrests, every form of disaster that might befall a community, and even the crash of technology requiring a return to manual systems. All of this simulation modeling has several objectives: minimizing the negative impact from a situation, improving response capacity, and developing psychological resilience in the face of adversity. Those skills that have guided our clinical practice can easily be transformed into leadership resilience.

Psychological resilience is the capacity to respond quickly and constructively to adversity, whether in the form of an actual crisis or a perceived disappointment. As we know through simulating the response to adverse clinical outcomes, resilience capacity can be coached and developed with practice. The first step in the process, supported by decades of research in psychology, is to develop an understanding of our distinct and often unconscious pattern for dealing with adversity. Margolis and Stoltz (2010) have identified four lenses through which managers can effectively view adverse events to create a shift toward what they refer to as a *resilience* regimen:

- **Control:** When a crisis hits, do you look for opportunities for immediate improvement rather than identifying all of the contributory factors—even those beyond your control?

- **Impact:** Are you able to avoid the temptation to look for the origins of the problem in yourself or others and focus instead on identifying what positive effects your actions might have?

- **Breadth:** Do you assume that the underlying cause of a crisis is specific and able to be contained rather than defaulting to thinking it will cast a pall over your career?

- **Duration:** How long do you assume the crisis and its aftermath will last?

(Margolis & Stoltz, 2010, p. 88)

The first two points characterize your personal reaction to adversity and the second two your impression of the magnitude. By understanding all four, you will begin to assess your current response to challenges, setbacks, and failures as the backdrop to develop better adversity coping skills. The goal is to create a shift in your personal beliefs, resulting in an improved ability to lead an organization through adversity while maintaining positive self-esteem and confidence.

This change in mind-set can be practiced by changing the lens through which the situation is first viewed. Rather than engaging in cause-oriented thinking, Margolis and Stoltz (2010) suggest the more productive response orientation. Table 6.1 illustrates the difference.

TABLE 6.1 Productive Response Orientation

CAUSE-ORIENTED THINKING	RESPONSE-ORIENTED THINKING
CONTROL Was this adverse event inevitable, or could I have prevented it?	What features of the situation can I (even potentially) improve?
IMPACT Did I cause the adverse event, or did it result from external forces?	What sort of positive impact can I personally have on what happens next?
BREADTH Is the underlying cause of this event specific to it or more widespread?	How can I contain the negatives of the situation and generate currently unseen positives?
DURATION Is the underlying cause of this event enduring or temporary?	What can I do to begin addressing the problem now?

Reprinted from Margolis & Stoltz, 2010

The risky and unstable corporate environment that requires a CEO to be able to see around corners suggests that adaptability will provide the much-needed competitive edge. The traditional approaches to strategy execution assume a relatively stable world where a competitive advantage is typically built on brand stability, dominating a market, exploiting certain capabilities, or occupying a unique niche. Consider for a moment, however, that McDonald's has become the largest seller of coffee in the United Kingdom. In a stable business environment, would we have imagined that the world's largest seller of fast food burgers could ever become a global contender in coffee sales? Yet these types of market shifts are occurring in health care in markets once considered predictable and where the big players controlled a substantial percentage of the market share.

Reeves and Deimler (2011) claim that management adaptability is really composed of two distinct features: the ability to quickly and accurately read the signals in the market and then to quickly mobilize to take bold action. In order to adapt, CEOs must have their antennae tuned to signals of change in the environment, decode those signals, and quickly act to reinvent business models or even reshape the market. The authors reference the sport of auto racing as an example of adapting to change through processing complex signals. Contemporary racing automobiles are equipped with hundreds of sensors on critical engine and body parts. These sensors collect and process data on everything from road conditions to weather and, when run through sophisticated simulators, guide course corrections in real time. Our industry requires similarly precise course corrections based on timely analysis of data and creative actions based on this information.

In order to fully understand these complex problems, we need to become adept at mining, manipulating, and analyzing big data. McKinsey defines big data as data sets with sizes beyond the ability of commonly used software tools to capture, curate, manage, and process the data (Manyika et al., 2011). Because the amount of data in our world has been exploding, analyzing large data sets will become a key basis of competition, underpinning new waves of productivity growth, innovation, and consumer surplus, according to research by MGI and McKinsey's Business Technology Office (Manyika et al., 2011). Leaders in every sector will have to grapple with the implications of big data, not just a few data-oriented managers. The increasing volume and detail of information captured by enterprises, the rise of multimedia, social media, and the Internet of Things will fuel exponential growth in data for the foreseeable future (Manyika et al., 2011).

CEOs in industries worldwide are leveraging this signal reading to bypass slow-moving decision hierarchies and make real-time adjustments to strategy and operations, staying ahead of the curve and financially viable. These data, specifically consumer response to these interventions, provide the basis for experimentation with new products and services. Whereas in the past we made decisions based on averages and feedback was provided at glacial speed, we can now use detailed customer data to generate, simulate, and replicate more complex ideas faster and at lower costs. This will support an environment that encourages knowledge flow, diversity, autonomy, sharing, risk-taking, and the flexibility upon which adaptation thrives (Reeves & Deimler, 2011).

Like no time in the past, the disruptive players—the mavericks—will set the pace for innovation. The CEO who follows market trends, focuses on countering the positions taken by competitors, or succumbs to the slow-moving organizational hierarchy will be left behind. The competitive advantage will be earned by the CEO with the ability to address uncertainty head on, quickly examine the risks and create initiatives to confront each opportunity, utilize sound data to manage the execution of the plan, and do so with speed and boldness—in other words, gain the ability to see around corners with 20/20 vision.

What Is Holding You Back?

So you want to get to the corner office, whether in a hospital, health care, educational, or entrepreneurial setting. What's holding you back? What is keeping you from achieving the success for which you feel you are prepared? It could be a number of things.

Over the years Connie and I have observed nurses in a variety of settings who were bright, patient-centered, well-educated individuals who had much to contribute but had not yet achieved—and maybe never would achieve—their goals. Why? A number of reasons. Take a deep breath and consider whether any of these things may be contributing to your inability to rise beyond your current role.

The Way You Look

Years ago the traditional attire for nurses was starched white uniforms with distinctive white hats. Those days are long gone; today's nurses wear a wide range of uniforms guided in some cases by the policies of the places where they work and in others by their own personal preferences. Those in clinical positions are certainly hampered in terms of what they can wear; those in administrative positions are not so hampered. In both areas we have seen attire that, frankly, holds people back:

- Wild designs and crazy colors on scrubs; cartoon themes may be appropriate in a pediatric ward but not in an emergency department.

- "Trendy" hairstyles.

- Visible tattoos.

Jaworek (2001) examined what constituted acceptable modern office attire and whether casually dressed women were perceived as serious about their work or career (this applies to men as well). Her opinion (and ours): no! The situation today is no different. If you want to be perceived as someone who belongs in the corner office, you must dress and present yourself as though you belong in the corner office. The top executives we interviewed *looked* like top executives. Do you?

How You Interact With Others

The nurse executives we interviewed strongly pointed to the ability to interact well with others as a key factor in their own success; we agree.

Nurses, says Pat O'Donoghue, must learn how to work with people and how to motivate them. "You gain those skills every day whether interacting with a patient, a doctor, a colleague, or whomever," she says. "One of the things that nurses learn early on is good communication skills, which is fundamental. You have to listen to what people are trying to tell you, their body language, and pay total attention during these interactions. Another skill nurses must master is how to communicate your own ideas. Without mastering these areas, success is not attainable."

Leadership, by its very nature, involves working with and through other people. It requires the ability to gain consensus over sometimes contentious issues. It requires the ability to influence others in positive ways to perform effectively in the pursuit of mutual goals. Leadership requires followership; you can't achieve followership if you do not interact effectively with others.

"You cannot underestimate the power of simply being around," says Paula Lucey. "I make rounds quite a bit. Being visible is very important—to me it's all about relationships. You need to go out and talk to folks whether you're talking to them and using the Studer method of very structured rounds or you're just walking around and saying, 'Oh, how's it going today?', or 'I really like your outfit today.'"

The Ability to See the "Big Picture"

Nurses can hold themselves back by failing to see the forest for the trees—by being overly focused on their little corner of the world and not understanding the broader issues that impact the organization as a whole. Successful executives have learned to move beyond a small focus on a clinical area—or even the nursing profession—as Rhonda Anderson points out.

As a nurse in a CEO role, she says, "Your nurse colleagues tend to have you in a spotlight or a fishbowl and really are watching what you're doing and whether you're advocating for them." But, she notes, that's not the role of the CEO, even a nurse CEO.

"Your role is to make sure that this organization, whether it is a multihospital group, a single hospital, or whatever it might be, has a strategy for business development, that it knows exactly its role in the community, that it has an overall understanding of what is going on, locally and nationally, from a political and public policy standpoint so that those things can all be aligned." Without this broad perspective, she says, "you will sink the boat. And, obviously you can't be in that role and sink the boat."

In your current role, you may be focused on meeting the needs of the patients you serve or employees you manage. As you rise to progressively higher levels within your organization, you must find a balance between meeting the needs of those you now serve and meeting the needs of the broader organization—and its communities. Finding this balance can be challenging, but it is critical in your rise within your organization or profession.

Getting the "big picture" means having a clear understanding of the mission and vision of the organization. It means moving beyond the need and desire to "help and protect" your position, role, or profession toward an understanding that sometimes tough decisions (i.e., decisions that may balance cost and quality) must be made and recognizing your role in supporting those decisions.

Additional Areas of Focus

Here are some additional areas you might consider as you assess your strengths and areas of opportunity to position yourself for increasingly more challenging roles:

- **Are your expectations realistic?** Your colleagues who are "part of the inner circle" know that they had to *earn* their way to this position—it is not a position that is simply conferred because of your position or title. Think of the executives in your organization. Some of them are more involved in decisions, more "players" than others. It has nothing to do with their titles; they earned those titles because of their positive traits and qualities.

- **Do you have a collaborative approach?** Leaders are often competitive, but successful leaders know that collaboration, not competition, is the best way to move ahead. Competing head-on with colleagues may get you what you are looking for in the short term, but in the long run, working with others to achieve results will have a greater positive impact on your career. Your goal should never be to "get my way." Your goal should be to "do the right thing."

- **Do you have an inclusive attitude?** Every relationship in your organization is important. Do not focus your efforts on nurturing relationships only with those whom you view to be in "important" positions. There is much to gain—professionally and personally—by forming relationships with a broad variety of individuals, from frontline staff, to part-timers, to managers and CEOs. Each relationship provides you with a new perspective and a greater understanding of the issues that affect your organization. That understanding can help you make better recommendations and will build your reputation as someone who has a broad, strategic perspective.

- **Is your focus based more on facts than feelings?** This can be tough for nurses to do, but if you want to become a successful and respected leader, you need to make sure that your recommendations are based on facts—not feelings. Your opinions are valid only to the extent that they are based on practical experience or hard data.

- **Do you have a proactive approach?** Do you sense that you are left out of decisions that you could contribute to? Are you frustrated that nobody ever asks you for your opinions? There is a simple solution: *Ask* to be included. Too many people assume that their superiors know that they would like to be included or know that they have knowledge and information that could be helpful to the organization. They give their superiors too much credit. Chances are they *do not* know. You need to tell them. Chances are that a lot of people in your organization who are involved and whose opinions are valued did not sit back and wait for someone to invite them to participate. They asked for the opportunity. You should too.

When you consider your career goals and your current position, what is holding you back? It may be challenging for you to tell. If you frequently wonder why your ideas are met with indifference or why you just do not get the respect you feel you "deserve," you may be lacking awareness of some specific traits or behaviors that may be affecting others' perceptions of you.

What to do? Mentors can be a good source of input, as we have discussed. Another option might be to connect with a career counselor who can assess your strengths and offer a third-party perspective on areas where you may need to make changes to present a more polished, professional brand.

If a professional career coach is not an option, you may want to rely on the advice and counsel of a trusted friend or colleague.

Ask for some direct and candid feedback. Then be open to what you hear. Too often we have a tendency to make excuses or discount the feedback we receive. But if you are willing to open yourself up to feedback that may be difficult to hear, you will be making the first step to personal improvement.

While sometimes we self-identify areas that we can either strengthen or improve, in other cases we learn through feedback from others. In fact, the process of actively seeking out feedback—positive and constructive—is an important best practice that all of our executive nurses identified, and they all pointed to various mentors who gave them feedback and counseling along their way to the corner office.

Executive Leadership Lessons

- The traits of extroversion, emotional stability, agree-ableness, conscientiousness, and openness to experi-ence are highly correlated with success.

- Demographic, human capital, motivational, and orga-nizational variables explained significant variance in objective career success and career satisfaction; most notably, the educational level, quality, prestige, and degree type all predicted financial success.

- Underpinning all of these traits was the need for flexibility and balance—being flexible to address the myriad opportunities and challenges that will come your way and finding a way to balance competing demands of personal and professional priorities.

- A CEO must balance the agility required to thrive amidst the chaos with the need to create a culture where employees and other stakeholders are secure and confident and able to successfully execute the goals of the organization.

- Recovering from adversity is a requisite skill of the corner office executive.

- Develop an understanding of your distinct and often unconscious pattern for dealing with adversity, and build capacity for managing chaos and adversity.

- Management adaptability is composed of two distinct features: the ability to quickly and accurately read the signals in the market and then to quickly mobilize to take bold action.

- Create an environment that encourages knowledge flow, diversity, autonomy, sharing, risk-taking, and the flexibility upon which adaptation thrives.

- Leaders are often competitive, but successful leaders know that collaboration, not competition, is the best way to move ahead.

- Ask to be included in corporate decision-making—do not wait to be asked.

- Be a data-driven decision-maker; be sure that your ideas and recommendations are based on facts—not feelings. Your opinions are valid only to the extent that they are based on practical experience or hard data.

- Understand the broader issues facing the organization; do not focus on your corner of the world exclusively.

- If you want to be perceived as someone who belongs in the corner office, you must dress and present yourself as though you belong in the corner office.

References

Barrick, M. R., & Mount, M. K. (1991). The big five personality dimensions and job performance: A meta-analysis. *Personnel Psychology, 44*(1), 1-26.

Buckingham, M., & Clifton, D.O. (2001). *Now, discover your strengths*. New York, NY: The Free Press.

Clark, D. (2011). Reinventing your personal brand. *Harvard Business Review, 89*(3), 78-81.

Farson, R., & Keyes, R. (2002). The failure-tolerant leader. *Harvard Business Review, 80*(8), 64-71.

Jaworek, J. (2001). Too clothes for comfort? *Incentive, 175*(10), 40-41.

Judge, T. A., Cable, D. M., Boudreau, J. W., & Bretz, Jr., R. D. (1995). An empirical investigation of the predictors of executive career success. *Personnel Psychology, 48*(3), 485-519.

Longfellow, H. W. (n.d.). Retrieved from http://www.brainyquote. com/quotes/authors/h/henry_wadsworth_longfello.html

Manyika, J., Chui, M., Brown, B., Bughin, J., Dobbs, R., Roxburgh, C., & Byers, A. H. (2011). *Big data: The next frontier for innovation, competition, and productivity*. Retrieved October 22, 2012, from http://www.mckinsey.com/Insights/MGI/ Research/Technology_and_Innovation/Big_data_The_next_ frontier_for_innovation

Margolis, J. D., & Stoltz, P. G. (2010). How to bounce back from adversity. *Harvard Business Review, 88*(1), 86-92.

Quorum Health Resources. (2011). *Hospital trustee quick reference guide*. Brentwood, CA: QHR Learning Institute.

Reeves, M., & Deimler, M. (2011). Adaptability: The new competitive advantage. *Harvard Business Review, 89*(7/8), 134-414.

Chapter 7
Credentials, Clubs, and Contacts

"I understood the need to connect professionally, and, while I had been a member of ASMSA while I was with Emory, I had not transitioned off 'Emory's registry' for being a member to HCA. So I called and asked if I could be a member and was told, 'No—you're a for-profit.' But I filled out all the forms anyway, and I sent them in. They sent me a letter telling me I could not be a member because I did not have 'line authority over a practice'—at that time we had something like 140 hospitals! That's when I learned that you had to understand how to work the circuit. Because I got on the phone and I called Connie; I called all of these other people and before I knew it, I was in."
–Roy Simpson, September 2012

Credentials do make a difference, and, without exception, the nurses we interviewed have pursued various forms of education to further both their personal interests and their professional careers. Some started out with the desire to attain high levels of education; others found academia through less direct pursuits. All recall with fondness their alma maters and the many people who influenced them throughout their careers.

Some, like Connie, wish they had taken a different path. Connie acknowledges that she has few regrets when it comes to her career, but if there was one, it was that she would have gone to "better schools."

What Credentials and From Where?

"My undergraduate from Wisconsin was fabulous," Connie says. "My master's at DePaul, at the time, was one of the most progressive in the country, and it served me very well." It is her doctorate she wishes she would have approached differently. "I checked into the University of Chicago in organizational behavior and it was really, really expensive, and I could go to the state school for next to nothing; so I went to the state school for next to nothing." She was, at the time, in her early 20s, so cost was a significant factor. Looking back, though, she says, "Because I was so young, that educational theory was going to have to last me." In hindsight, she would have invested more. Later in life, she would pursue a 3-year program at Harvard that was both expensive and valuable, she says. "I learned a lot, and the connections and the networking and the global thing were wonderful."

Pat Thompson's educational pursuits were driven by geography, she recalls. As the child of a military family, Pat found herself moving frequently, and when it came time to choose a college, she wanted to select one near a family member. She chose Louisiana because her grandmother lived there. "I went to my grandmother and said, 'Find me a college near you that has a nursing program.'" She applied and was accepted at Northwestern State University in Louisiana and attended the main campus in Natchitoches and then the clinical campus in Shreveport.

Later, when she went on to pursue her master's degree at the urging of a faculty mentor, she chose to go to the University of Alabama in Birmingham, which was near her sister. When she graduated, she went immediately into teaching and later enrolled in graduate school while working full time and shortly after adopting her 3-year-old daughter. Ultimately she received her doctorate in nursing administration with a minor in business management.

For nurses in today's environment, credentials matter—not only for nurses, but also for the patients they serve. American Nurses Association (ANA) President Karen Daley says, "It is critically important that nurses without a BSN take advantage of opportunities to pursue advanced education in order to become better prepared to care for patients in an increasingly complex heath care delivery system" (Daley, 2011, p. 3).

Daley is not alone in her thinking, of course. In *The Future of Nursing: Leading Change, Advancing Health,* the Institute of Medicine (IOM, 2010) shares four key messages developed through the work of the Committee on the Robert Wood Johnson Foundation Initiative, which was launched in 2008 to conduct a 2-year analysis to respond to the need to assess and transform the nursing profession. The committee's four key messages included:

- Nurses should practice to the full extent of their education and training.

- Nurses should achieve higher levels of education and training through an improved education system that promotes seamless academic progression.

- Nurses should be full partners, with physicians and other health care professionals, in redesigning health care in the United States.

- Effective workforce planning and policymaking require better data collection and information infrastructure. (IOM, 2010)

Peggy Ward-Smith, PhD, RN (2011), points back to a 1965 position paper from the ANA that stated that a baccalaureate degree (BSN) should be the minimum requirement for entry into nursing and looks forward to continued emphasis on the critical importance of highly educated nurses. She makes the case for the importance of effectively educating nurses to provide higher-quality, safer, more affordable, and more accessible care and says that she would like to see the IOM's recommendations tied to some consequences. "Requiring places of employment to oblige graduates of ADN and diploma programs to return to school within an acceptable time frame after obtaining licensure—perhaps 5 years—is one potential intervention" (Ward-Smith, 2011, p. 10). Furthermore, "The nurse with a BSN should be financially rewarded for his or her education" (Ward-Smith, 2011, p. 10). Without these consequences, she predicts, the IOM recommendation may go as far as the ANA's recommendation in 1965.

Ellenbecker (2010) agrees with this approach: "Today's environment of expanding knowledge, the call for interdisciplinary healthcare delivery teams, and evidence of the relationship between nurse education and improved patient outcomes strongly indicate the need for nurses prepared at the baccalaureate level. Requiring a baccalaureate degree for entry into nursing practice, and as the initial degree of nursing education would prepare nurses earlier for graduate education and the much needed roles of educator, researcher and advanced practice nurse. The nursing profession should take the lead in advocating for educational policies that would adequately prepare the nurse workforce of the future" (p. 115).

Clearly, those nurses who choose to pursue higher education will find themselves in the enviable position of not only being highly valued by health care and other organizations, but will be contributing to the need to ensure high levels of quality to meet the needs of patients.

But education, of course, is just part of the picture. Nurses must remain relevant throughout their careers, even after their formal education has been completed. Participation in professional organizations can help provide this relevancy, as well as valuable connections.

Which Organizations and Why?

There are a wide range of nursing organizations that can provide value for nurses in today's rapidly changing health care landscape:

- The American College of Healthcare Executives (ACHE; http://www.ache.org) is an international professional society with more than 40,000 members representing executives at hospitals, health care systems, and other health care organizations. The organization offers fellow of the ACHE (FACHE) accreditation, which is highly sought after and well recognized among health care leaders.

- The ANA (http://www.nursingworld.org) offers continuing professional development and certification, in addition to resources ranging from webinars to conferences.

- The American Organization of Nurse Executives (AONE; http://www.aone.org) is the national organization of nurses who design, facilitate, and manage care. A subsidiary of the American Hospital Association, the AONE provides leadership, professional development, advocacy, and research to advance nursing practice and patient care, promote nursing leadership excellence, and shape public policy for health care.

- The Healthcare Financial Management Association (http://www.hfma.org) develops and promotes ethical, high-quality health care finance practices and has more than 39,000 members.

- Rotary International (http://www.rotary.org) is a community-based service club whose mission is to bring together business and professional leaders to provide humanitarian services, encourage high ethical standards in all vocations, and help build goodwill and peace in the world. There are about 35,000 clubs with more than 1.2 million members worldwide.

- Sigma Theta Tau International (http://www.nursing society.org), an honor society, supports the learning, knowledge, and professional development of nurses committed to making a difference in health worldwide.

- The U.S. Chamber of Commerce (http://www.uscha ber.com) is a national business federation that works to create a favorable climate for business in the United States and around the world. In addition to the national group, there are many local groups around the country; any community can organize and support a chamber of commerce.

- The Young Presidents' Organization (YPO; http:// www.ypo.org) is a network of more than 20,000 chief executives leading companies based in 120 countries. Members must be under the age of 45 years and be a chief operator of a company that meets minimum size and revenue requirements (upon turning 50 years of age, members may transition to the World Presidents' Organization).

P. K. Scheerle has had experience with the YPO. In fact, she was the first woman in Louisiana to be part of this group in the early 1990s. It was, she says, an opportunity to both learn and to teach. "I went to everything they offered and, like anything, you get out of it what you put into it," she says. She adds, "As a leader in the YPO, I saw men that needed more of an understanding of what a woman could contribute in a boardroom or at the top of the organization—and I was always quick to offer that help to those individuals who needed it."

Her involvement in this organization, she says, "gave me the confidence to realize that I had a gift and, if I didn't use it to strengthen this worthy profession of nursing to be a powerhouse in health care, I was wasting my life."

Paula Lucey notes that both the Robert Wood Johnson nurse executive program and the Johnson & Johnson Wharton program (which no longer exists) were both extremely helpful for her. The Johnson & Johnson program, she says, "really taught me a lot about system and looking at things from a system perspective." That was back in 1995. "At that time, it was revolutionary. It really pushed me from being a manager to being a leader—to really look at the big picture and the system."

There are, quite literally, thousands of organizations that can provide nurses with the opportunity to both learn and teach. Associations exist for every specialty in nursing and for nursing avocations as well. A search online for nursing associations will yield more than 5 million results. In addition to the traditional associations, today's wired environment also provides ample opportunity for nurses to connect with each other virtually. On LinkedIn, arguably the most professionally oriented of the popular social media sites, there are more than 1,400 groups focused on aspects of the nursing profession. The largest among them are the Nursing Network (21,000+ members), The R.N. Network-Nursing Careers (9,000+ members), Nursing Beyond the Bedside (5,000+ members), and Nursing Jobs (8,800). Nurses engaging in these groups can build their networks and enhance their expertise through interaction and sharing.

Networking is, in fact, an often-mentioned element of nurses' rise to the top. Importantly, contacts need to be managed and nurtured to keep them valuable.

The Care and Feeding of Your Contacts

Building a strong network is about more than simply developing a network; strong networks require nurturing. The principle of reciprocity comes into play here—the idea that relationships are built based on mutual gain. That gain may take the form of simply enjoying to be in another's company, or it may be based on some other value that the relationship provides. In business settings, many of the relationships we established are based upon the value that we may receive from others because of their experience and insights—or their own contacts. Importantly, though, successful leaders learn that they must give more than they get.

Even those in the early stages of their careers can provide value to their more seasoned colleagues. They may be more knowledgeable about the use of technology or social media; they may have valuable perspectives about what their generation is looking for in terms of a rewarding career experience.

As you build your network, you should also be thinking about how you can give and gain value from that network. This might mean nominating your contacts for jobs, recognition, or honors in their field of activity or areas of interest. It might mean sending them information about topics in which they have expressed an interest or about issues they are currently addressing. It might mean clipping an item from a trade or professional journal where you saw their name or organization mentioned. It might be inviting them for coffee or lunch from time to time. The key is to find ways to provide value to your contacts through their relationship to you. Basically you want to keep your name in front of them so that they are also thinking of you when they hear of issues, information, jobs, or other opportunities that may crop up.

One thing that Connie has done to keep her name in front of her large list of contact is to send out Thanksgiving cards instead of the more common holiday card. "I didn't want to get lost in all of the other holiday cards, and I really wanted to communicate my thankfulness," she says.

Today, of course, social media has provided us with the ability to connect with more people more quickly and more frequently than ever before. Tools such as Facebook, Twitter, LinkedIn, and Google+ are specifically designed to build networks of individuals with shared interests, vocations, and avocations.

LinkedIn is Therese's go-to social media tool, because she finds that it has particular relevance for business professionals. It also has some great online opportunities for networking and building credibility and expertise. LinkedIn is one of the more "business oriented" of the social media sites, and one of the tools it offers is "groups." There are literally thousands of groups covering interests ranging from Anesthesia Professionals (2,928 members) to a group for those interested in zoonotics (Rabies Management Group, with 73 members). There are groups that can help you both learn and leverage your career interests and talents.

You are able to join up to 50 groups; the more groups you join, the more people to whom you are potentially connected, which expands your ability both to be noticed through others' online searches and to have more access to others when you are searching for information or hoping to make new contacts.

An important point when selecting groups in which to participate: Size does not really matter. Very large groups can provide you with access to many people and viewpoints and enhance your network, but smaller groups can be more focused and yield richer discussions and opportunities for interaction. There are three ways to find groups that might be of interest, notes Jan Vermeiren, founder of Networking Coach, a LinkedIn training company and the author of *How to Really Use LinkedIn* (2009). Vermeiren indicates three ways to find groups that might be of interest:

1. **Through the groups directory.** The box at the top right-hand side of your LinkedIn home page that will allow you to search for people, updates, jobs, companies, and groups.

2. **Through similar groups.** Once you join a group LinkedIn will provide you with a list of similar groups you may be interested in.

3. **Through others' profiles.** Check the profiles of those to whom you are connected or those you admire to see which groups they belong to, and check them out.

In terms of participation in groups, it is really much like traditional face-to-face networking:

- First listen, then talk. Do not start your own discussions until you have gotten a sense for the "culture" of the group.

- Select the right groups for you based on your professional and personal interests.

- Never sell in a group—that is a sure way to turn people off.

If you do a search on LinkedIn, you will find groups for all of the major nursing and business associations and every type of clinical practice or interest you might imagine. Here are some additional LinkedIn groups that you may want to consider as you work to build your network exponentially online:

Group: Healthcare Executive.net
Created: 2008
Members: 26,000
About: A real-time network of C-level through middle management-level health care executives, including medical, acute care, pharmaceutical, long-term care, nursing, pharmacy, specialized, and related field professionals.

Group: Nurse Entrepreneurs
Created: 2008
Members: 6,500
About: A group for nurse entrepreneurs or those wanting to be nurse entrepreneurs.

Group: Nursing Beyond the Bedside
Created: 2010
Members: 5,000
About: A community of nurses working in, or interested in, nonbedside/nonclinical nursing, including nurse case management, utilization review, appeals/denials, clinical documentation improvement, risk management, Healthcare Effectiveness Data and Information Set (HEDIS), medical record review, nurse informatics, nurse educator, and any nursing professional in a nonbedside role.

Group: Nursing Network
Created: 2008
Members: 21,000
About: A group dedicated to networking nursing professionals and others associated with the nursing profession.

Group: Nursing Professionals
Created: 2008
Members: 4,900
About: A group to bring together nursing professionals for networking purposes. All nurses and those pursuing nursing as a career are welcome to join. It is not open to recruitment companies and others wishing to sell to nurses.

Finding the Right Mentor

Contacts are important, but mentors are invaluable. Some of the most successful people across multiple professions point to relationships with mentors as the springboard to their personal and professional success: musicians, sports figures, actors, and, yes, businesspeople, often point to others who have provided them with critical perspectives and served as personal consultants, professional critics, and friendly advisors. They may be business or personal contacts. They may be older or younger than you (in fact, a trend toward "reverse-mentoring" is emerging as a by-product of our increasingly technology-driven world). Importantly, they do not necessarily need to come from your own profession, industry, geography, or background. In fact, it can be better if they do not.

Mentoring relationships are sometimes set up formally through organizations or associations in which we work. But informal relationships are formed all of the time, and you should not hesitate to be proactive in seeking mentors.

As Pat Thompson said to us, "So many times, people think that you have to wait for somebody to come to you to be a mentor. There's no rule that says you can't get a mentor. I say more than one, because you have mentors for different skill sets or across time or one that's pretty long-term and others that are short-term. This whole concept of mentors is not a one-size-fits-all, and it is perfectly OK to identify someone you know and respect, or even someone you might not know. It's the idea of realizing that it's really important to take that responsibility and to know that it's OK for you to find a mentor. Most people, I think, would actually be pretty honored and willing to help if somebody came up and said to them, 'I have seen your work; I have wanted your work; I so respect how you do things, and you have some skill sets that I really would like to develop, and I would appreciate some help to develop if you have the time.'"

Thompson recommends finding some trusted friends or colleagues who will tell you the truth as you are working through an issue or as you are trying to develop or do something—people who will give you honest, constructive feedback. "When you're in a CEO position, not many people will do that for you," she says. "They don't want to insult you, and so you really need a core group of a few folks you can trust and talk with and also get some really solid, honest feedback from."

Therese recalls that she has had many mentors along the way. "I have been blessed with the best mentors that anyone could have, and I have relied on them for different things. I had a mentor early in my career who was the world's best communicator, and she helped me to sort of round out my rough edges in terms of communication—how to get a message across in a way that my message could be heard in a more productive, positive way."

Connie has also relied on mentors throughout her career and still does today. "If I saw people that did something particularly well, I wanted to make a connection with them and learn from them," she says. "I've done that often. The man who was CFO at Montefiore was just so smart about money and so smart about financial strategy that he really helped me move into a whole new way of thinking about how to leverage your assets and how to leverage finances.

"Warren Buffett doesn't know it, but I think he's my mentor in some ways. It's about trying to find people who do things particularly well and trying to learn from them. I still do that all the time, formally and informally. When I was at Harvard for a training session recently, one of my favorite professors from 10 years ago was there—I'm still learning from him."

Lois Zachary, EdD, is the author of *The Mentor's Guide* and *Creating a Mentoring Culture* and the president of Leadership Development Services LLC in Phoenix. Multiple mentoring relationships are important to allow us to gather wisdom from multiple sources, says Zachary (2011). When seeking mentors, Zachary emphasizes the importance of looking for those who are *not* like you. The natural tendency, she says, is for mentors to be selected based on "chemistry." Instead, she says, it is important to consider:

- Whether the potential mentor will challenge your thinking and encourage you to constantly raise the bar for personal growth and development.

- Whether the potential mentor has the expertise, experience, time, and willingness to help achieve your desired learning goals.

- Whether you will feel comfortable learning from this individual; is there a "good learning fit"? (Zachary, 2011)

Forming a mentoring relationship is not about walking up to someone and saying, "Will you be my mentor?," although that happens. Instead, say something like, "Would you be willing to meet with me a couple of times over the next few months? I'd like to tell you a little bit about myself, and I feel there's a lot I could learn from you. Would you have the time for that?"

Today, of course, mentoring relationships do not need to exist in "real time" or even involve face-to-face contact. Connections can take place in "virtual space." That truly expands the ability of nursing professionals to cast a wide net when seeking mentors, and the Internet makes this easier than ever to do through tools like LinkedIn, which are designed to help nurture professional networking relationships, literally around the world.

A tool that Zachary (2011) recommends is the "personal board of directors." Using this model, "an individual seeks out and recruits multiple mentors to help achieve specific goals," she says. Under the model, mentors meet with the mentee at regular intervals. It is up to the mentee to manage the learning process by making calls and hosting the meetings. That way, both mentor and mentee share accountability for the learning process and achieving the desired results.

For us, as well as for the nurse leaders we consulted in writing this book, those individuals we have looked to as mentors throughout our careers have been incredibly significant. Importantly, as we were mentored, so must we mentor others. As we recognize the experiences and mentorship that helped us get to the positions we are in now, we need to look backward and pull others along with us. Connie excels at that.

"Every single time she has moved into a new, interesting, innovative role, she looks behind her, reaches out her arms, and pulls up everyone in her circle into the next level that she has sort of left behind," says Therese. "You continue to sort of move in your career as Connie moves in hers into all sorts of interesting things. When she gets a phone call from someone who says, 'Connie, do you know a nurse that may . . .,' she looks to her circle or mentees and provides those experiences."

Pat O'Donoghue also says that giving back through mentoring has been important to her. "I do have that sense of obligation of trying to do exactly the same thing," she says. "I have an unfailing belief in the potential of every person to grow, to learn, and to make a contribution. My role is to understand how I can help them to achieve that goal."

Pat and other nurse leaders have always been quick to provide that support. In fact, Therese is part of a long-standing group of nurses who were her direct reports while she was the chief nursing officer (CNO) of a hospital in Milwaukee. "Two years ago, we had a sort of reunion of my nursing leadership team from that time," she recalls. "Every one of these individuals who were nurse managers at the time have gone on to become directors or CNOs. Everyone who was a director is now either a product line VP or an executive themselves."

The onus is on nurse leaders to provide that type of support and mentoring to those who will eventually fill our shoes. It is more than an obligation—it is a privilege.

Executive Leadership Lessons

- Go to the absolute best school you can.

- Get the best degrees you can.

- Prepare to be a lifelong learner.

- Take advantage of new networking opportunities allowed through social media.

- As you advance in your career, look for opportunities to mentor others.

References

Daley, K. (2011). Advanced nursing education is better for patients. *American Nurse, 43*(2), 3.

Ellenbecker, C. (2010). Preparing the nursing workforce of the future. *Policy, Politics & Nursing Practice, 11*(3), 115-125.

Institute of Medicine (IOM). (2010). *The future of nursing: Leading change, advancing health.* Washington, DC: The National Academies Press.

Vermeiren, J. (2009). *How to really use LinkedIn.* Charleston, SC: BookSurge Publishing.

Ward-Smith, P. (2011). Everything old is new again. *Urologic Nursing, 31*(1), 9-10.

Zachary, L. J. (2011). *The mentor's guide: Facilitating effective learning relationships* (2nd ed.). New York, NY: Jossey-Bass.

Chapter 8
Conclusion: Break Out of Your Limits

"About the trip to the corner office—why? Is someone looking for a title and a corner office, or are they looking to do the work that really needs to be done? Too often somebody says, 'I want to be (fill in the title),' not, 'I want to make this difference or provide this opportunity.' You need to figure out what you want and not what title you desire. It's quite simple—what makes you jump out of bed each morning, and what makes you pull the covers over your head? Make two lists, and when the next opportunity comes along, compare it to those two lists."

–Rhonda Anderson, September 2012

In examining the career paths of the corner office executives, a number of remarkable similarities emerged from their stories. From early in their student and professional lives, these executives deliberately managed their careers, seeking out the education and varied experiences that provided the foundation for positions of increasing scope and responsibility. These assertive executives worked tirelessly to achieve success, and along the way they developed the requisite competencies and the confidence to take on even more ambitious challenges at each turn. They never permitted themselves to fall victim to the winds of industry change or organizational whimsy, but rather, they stayed far ahead of the curve, thereby creating opportunities to add value in their corporations or to use those winds as the impetus to develop successful business models around new products and services. As Roy Simpson aptly stated, "The successful executive knows how to read the tea leaves. Being in this complex business world today, you can't be naïve." Their incremental and persistent successes fueled the confidence required to make increasingly bold decisions, take greater risks, and hone the predictive abilities required to shape their environments rather than simply participate in a world created by others. These executives were truly game changers.

Failure Is Not an Option

Early in their careers these executives distinguished themselves as trailblazers and experienced a number of firsts for their time: first woman to be accepted into an elite business organization, youngest member of a university faculty, college's first nurse president, first executive to be hired into a C-suite position while pregnant, or first nurse to sell a business to a particular venture capital firm. While each career was uniquely successful and profoundly gratifying for the executive, it would be naïve to presume that these risk-takers experienced careers that unfolded without a hitch. In fact, as fate usually dictates, every individual experiences some setbacks, disappointments, or even failures along the way: a much coveted position that went to another candidate, a missed business opportunity, or a decision made with timidity when bold action was required. Quite remarkably, each executive expressed difficulty in identifying career failures along the way. Perhaps more accurately stated, they had difficulty labeling an event as a disappointment or failure. "I remember the time when . . . no, I wouldn't call that a failure," or "I am hesitant to call that a failure because it really provided me the experience I needed for my following role," or "I may have held a position that I wasn't especially crazy about, but I would never think of it as a failure." One executive reported, "Sure I have been fired, but that gave me the opportunity to learn mergers and acquisitions and develop my career in a whole new direction."

While these successful executives are characteristically optimistic and resilient, they universally expressed the importance of "turning lemons into lemonade," or in business terms, assessing a situation, understanding the alternatives, mitigating the risk involved, and creating opportunity where disappointment seems the likely outcome. In their profound words, "I analyzed my failures or disappointments and extracted the key learnings." Several executives expressed similar thoughts, saying things like, "These learnings and experiences were then leveraged as my next success." Often this presented itself as an opening to take a greater risk in the future, because "if you have already seen the worst that can happen, you are less afraid to be bold. You know what failure looks like, so you know what to avoid, and you can therefore act with greater confidence. It makes you brave."

They all reported the exceptional ability to separate themselves from the event or situation when evaluating what may have gone wrong. In other words, they did not personalize the situation, permitting them the opportunity to objectively study events leading up to the disappointment or failure, assess the outcome, and immediately turn their learning into the next success. In addition to setting the stage for a more objective evaluation, they were also able to maintain the confidence of their organization as well as their self-confidence.

Several reported that a healthy balance of realism and optimism helped in maintaining perspective during these trying episodes. Organizations are highly complex environments and exist within an industry experiencing great tumult and where standard methods of operation are constantly challenged. In order to adapt to this fluctuating environment, these executives presumed that conflict, change, negotiation, and political dynamics would be their constant companions. Roy Simpson observed, "You will never get 100% of a situation from your vantage point, because it's a dynamic environment. You have to have good intuition and emotional intelligence and the ability to manage the landscape. Sure I've had some down times, but overall I am very excited to be a nurse; it's a great profession."

Successful executives navigate these waters by first understanding their own strengths and weaknesses through an honest self-appraisal. This process is enhanced through the feedback of a trusted colleague. This is the colleague or mentor who is committed to your success, who possesses the insight to offer a new perspective and to assist in identifying the lessons and opportunities often lost in the debris of a failed endeavor. For a number of the corner office executives, this straight-talking individual was someone outside of nursing, someone with experience running a large corporation, or an entrepreneur or financier able to provide advice about the realities of selling a product or service in the current economic climate. This individual has the ability to tell you that "it's a good idea, but the timing is wrong" or "it's a good idea, but investors will never go for it." It is important to remember that executive nurses are trailblazers and relative newcomers to the corner office; therefore, they are likely to benefit from the experience of executive mentors from industries outside of nursing. These are professionals with corner office experience and a willingness to point out landmines in the corporate landscape, as well as to provide pointers to avoid the most deadly mistakes and make it to the corner office relatively unscathed.

To a person, the corner office executives remarked that "your stakeholders deserve the best of you." This requires a personal development plan with aggressive timelines and a willingness to seek out mentors, teachers, and guides to assist in competency development as well as exposure to learning opportunities through new projects, assuming additional responsibilities, and expressing a willingness to move outside of one's comfort zone, including responsibilities outside of nursing.

Large multinational Fortune 500 companies invest significantly in the development of C-suite talent. For those individuals marked for executive leadership roles, this often means overseas assignments to learn foreign markets, global distribution channels, system integration, and general management under extraordinary conditions. It is also likely that these high-potential executives will rotate through midlevel and senior roles in all of the significant functions within the corporation—supply chain, manufacturing, marketing, and product engineering to name a few. Health care organizations are beginning to see the benefit of a similar approach in the development of their high-potential talent. A CEO or chief operating officer (COO) provides better informed leadership, makes smarter financial decisions, and negotiates better deals with key stakeholders after having benefited from a deep understanding of all of the organization's critical functions. It is therefore essential that nurses with corner office aspirations negotiate opportunities to manage all functions and departments within the enterprise, including plant and facilities, construction projects, community relationships, and medical staff functional areas.

An example of this is an approach taken by a large Midwestern integrated regional health care system with more than 1,500 employed physicians. In an effort to improve current management outcomes and as a means of grooming executives for positions of increasing responsibility, system leadership very deliberately moves midlevel executives to new positions every several years. Think of how you might manage differently if you knew a colleague would soon step into your role and take over where you left off. Might you be more inclined to finish projects, execute strategies more aggressively, and manage expenses with greater precision? And as these executives move into new positions with increasing responsibilities, their decisions will be better informed and their problem-solving more creative and robust given the breadth and depth of experience they bring to their new position.

These tactics suggest a new paradigm in our approach to the management of our careers, a change that arguably needs to begin early in our professional socialization. As we identify those rising stars within nursing, our leaders must consider the need to expose these up-and-comers to experiences outside of our discipline and, although this seems quite obvious, pause and consider the difficulty some organizations experience when moving a staff nurse from critical care to telemetry or from labor and delivery to postpartum. As leaders we must communicate the significance of these experiences to the overall development of the corner office apprentice, but of equal importance is the requirement to create systems, process, and an organizational culture that supports and encourages these intraprofessional opportunities.

Whether the CEO of a hospital, president of a university, or successful business owner, these corner office executives all shared a number of interesting personal characteristics and experienced a number of similar approaches to their career progression. They planned their careers in a thoughtful and deliberate manner, based on an intelligent but aggressive strategy to reach their goals. While these pragmatic leaders leveraged their nursing know-how and built the professional infrastructure with the skills and competencies required for success, they all acknowledged the necessity of leaving some room for serendipity—that interesting opportunity that could not have been anticipated yet presents a unique challenge or an unanticipated opening into a profitable business realm. As several mentioned, "You must own your career" and "You need to be strategic about your career but flexible enough to consider the great opportunity that comes your way."

Opportunity Knocks for the Young

One of the remarkable distinguishing factors in these storied careers is the fact that these executives moved deliberately and expeditiously to the corner office. Quite extraordinarily, each of the corner office nurses was tapped on the shoulder very early in his or her career to assume their first leadership position, oftentimes within 6 to 12 months of graduation and initial licensure. They demonstrated an aptitude for leadership that set them apart from their peers, and they soon found themselves being groomed for positions of increasing responsibilities. In several instances, these leadership abilities were identified by faculty while the executive nurse was still a student.

We often perpetuate the myth within our profession that one must "put in the time" as a staff nurse before considering or being considered for a management position. We presume that significant time at the bedside is a prerequisite for leadership, and paying one's dues through working a fair share of undesirable shifts and similar rites of passage are critical to professional development. Furthermore, it is often difficult for us to understand that an individual interested in a management career might step into that arena through a nursing pathway. Yet, we watch with growing frustration the young graduates of MHA and MBA programs transition from their student roles directly into administrative residencies, which will, in no time at all, groom them for senior-level management positions and a fast track to the C-suite. It is important to note that many pursue this career path without a clinical undergraduate or graduate degree.

It must be recognized that there is a growing number of bright individuals with the interest and aptitude to manage health care organizations, as demonstrated by the growing enrollment in MHA and MBA programs with an academic emphasis on health care leadership. These programs are producing young leaders educated as professional executives ready to step into roles as consultants, product line or department leaders, financial executives, strategists, and physician practice managers to name a few. All are roles for which nurses are profoundly qualified and capable if we choose to eliminate our self-imposed glass ceiling and embrace the notion that management is a legitimate career in and of itself and, when coupled with a nursing education, a powerful addition to the corner office.

A growing number of physicians are pursuing graduate education in business, which positions them to become executives for large medical groups or health care organizations—as policymakers, investors, pharmaceutical leaders, or consultants— or as executives for regulatory agencies. These physicians, many recent medical school graduates, have expressed an interest in the business of health care and are leveraging their clinical expertise and experience in the C-suite or at the board table.

While it seems obvious, it may be easy to overlook the fact that not every nurse wishes to practice clinically; the financially inclined might prefer a role as budget director or chief financial officer, the creative communicator might thrive as an advertising executive or CEO, and the technology-savvy nurse with entrepreneurial inclinations might start a consulting practice as an informaticist. It is critical to note that none of these roles requires a traditional career trajectory beginning with a prescribed number of years as a staff nurse followed by progressive middle management positions. In fact, each of the corner office executives commented that they are continually grateful for their nursing credentials and especially appreciative of the fact that they were able to choose any number of varied career paths within health care or peripheral to health care *because* they were a nurse. In other words, nursing is an influential and commanding profession providing a highly leverageable repertoire of competencies, perspectives, and skills required for success as an executive leader of any enterprise.

This observation has significant implications for both individuals entering the profession as well as those who mentor and supervise the novice nurse. We are graduating many more second-career nurses from our educational programs—those who have substantial education or an established career in another field and, for a variety of economic or professional reasons, have chosen to pursue a career in nursing. They often have the credentials, experience, and drive to combine their two fields of expertise, such as business or finance, along with nursing, in order to pursue an executive role. These talented rising stars will benefit from mentorship, professional executive coaching, and exposure to interesting and varied projects as they look to marry these skill sets in the health care environment.

No one can argue with the growing empirical data documenting the importance of new graduate orientation as related to job success, professional socialization, personal engagement, patient safety, and minimizing the expense of turnover. In fact, the Institute of Medicine's (2010) *The Future of Nursing: Leading Change, Advancing Health* suggests what many nursing leaders have purported for some time: that graduating nurses and the greater health care system would benefit from a residency not unlike those required in the medical education system. But in our rush to standardize the socialization of new nurses, we should not lose sight of the importance of adapting these programs to the individual needs and career aspirations of the novice. The corner office executives were the beneficiaries of mentored opportunities and encouragement in the early development of their burgeoning leadership talent. Leaders took a calculated risk in fast-tracking these young professionals, and had they not taken this risk, perhaps opportunities would have been lost if these nurses had been required to remain in standardized orientation programs without the benefit of a customized approach. Obviously, this was a different era in health care: Lengths of stay were counted in weeks instead of hours, models of care were different, and patient acuity was demonstrably different. Nonetheless, it behooves us as leaders to strive to create an environment that empowers those nurses ready to step away from the group and spread their management wings. It is incumbent upon us as leaders to hone our talent-scouting abilities and identify those diamonds in the rough, the intellectually curious, talented, assertive nurses who may not yet possess all of the abilities noted throughout this text, but with the investment of time and coaching, could be the organization's CEO or state's senator or the inventor of a much-needed new model of care.

Elite Performance Through Executive Coaching

Elite athletes accomplish amazing feats of physical strength and endurance, breaking records in exponential fashion. In fact, as recently witnessed in the 2012 summer Olympics held in London, England, "a total of 38 records were broken. Some were improved by a few milliseconds, while others were shattered in blistering new times" (Rosales, 2012, p. 1). George Dvorsky (2012), quoting Gavin Thompson in the online newsletter io9, commented that today's athletes would hardly resemble those from a century ago. The winner of the men's 5,000 meter in Beijing ran at a pace that won the 1,500 meter in 1908. The winner of the women's marathon would have won the men's race in 1908 by an entire half hour. Today's athletes benefit from technological advances in everything from sleeker, computer-designed Speedo swimming apparel and less turbulent pools to high-performance footwear for track and field events (Silver, 2012).

Though aided by advances in engineering and sports science, these accomplishments are principally attributable to the athletes themselves and the precision training and coaching that prepare them for peak competitive performance. Membership in the ranks of the elite requires discipline, dedication, and physical strength, all of which are honed though personalized coaching around specific outcomes. In fact, at the collegiate level of competition, athletes demonstrating an aptitude for world-class competition are afforded a coach to further hone their talents through a personalized regimen.

World-class athletes spend a significant portion of their time not perfecting primary skills, which they have long ago mastered, but in evolving those secondary skills that will enable the execution of the primary skills. Their coaching emphasis is on building endurance, flexibility, strength, power, and agility. In fact, athletic coach Greg Glassman (n.d.), the originator of the CrossFit fitness regimen practiced by many world class athletes alongside their primary sport, contends that fitness should be defined as meaningful and measurable functional movements leading to increased work capacity across broad time and modal domains. In addition to swimming endless laps in the pool, Olympic swimmers also lift weights, run endless miles, and flip truck tires end over end in an effort to build stamina, strength, and endurance.

The corner office executives all mentioned the influence of others in their professional development and preparation for the senior positions they now hold, particularly the financial expertise they gained. Many of these executives did not have the benefit of the formal executive coaching that has now become a mainstay in corporate succession planning and management development, but they all spoke to the importance of mentors and other sage executives in their journey to the C-suite.

Executive performance specialist Tom Lemanski (n.d.), states that organizations typically hire for skills and knowledge, then promote on the basis of attitudes and habits. In an attempt to improve performance, they spend time and money developing the skills and knowledge; however, terminations typically occur from factors related to attitudes and habits.

Michelman (2004) reports that scores of major companies have made coaching a core part of executive development with the belief that under the right circumstances, one-on-one interaction with an objective third party can provide a focus that other forms of organizational support simply cannot. In fact, at the time of publication, IBM had more than 60 certified coaches among its ranks. While this level of intense coaching was once viewed as a tool to help correct underperformance, it is now more widely used to support top producers. In a white paper entitled *Linking Coaching to Business Results,* by Stephen Cohen of Right Management Consultants in Philadelphia (2009), 86% of companies surveyed reported that they used coaching to sharpen the skills of individuals who have been identified as future organizational leaders.

As one rises in the executive ranks, there is an increasing demand for results, and sadly, many executives receive scant and often unreliable performance feedback. As a result, many executives plateau in critical interpersonal and leadership skills. James Hunt (Hunt & Weintraub, 2011), of Babson College and author of *The Coaching Manager,* states that coaching is most effective when you know what you want to get done. Perhaps in spite of a stellar track record, the manager has not yet gained the interpersonal dexterity required of senior managers; that is, he or she is not yet a "black belt" in the art of influence, which is so important in the contemporary networked organization.

Rather than viewing coaching as performance remediation, nurses with their sights on the corner office should recognize that, just like the collegiate athlete with tremendous potential to succeed on the world stage, their organization is making a significant investment of time and money in developing their secondary skills. Such nurses will have honed their repertoire of clinical management competencies: outcomes management; safety and risk management; and staff, patient, and physician engagement. In fact, these competencies will be a welcomed and much needed addition to the organization's strategic planning, program development, and community accountability. These are the primary skills nurses bring to their executive role. Arguably, additional core skills, including strategic planning, financial skills, governance, and strategic human resources, will be required, but much like the Olympic athlete, the secondary skills—our corporate version of stamina, flexibility, power, and agility—need to be developed in order to assure success in the C-suite.

The Heart of a Leader

The difficult and circuitous route to the corner office is not for the faint of heart. Executives who strike out on a road not well traveled by nurses must possess a great degree of self-confidence and internal fortitude. In their words, there are several must-have characteristics that will make the journey not only easier but also more enjoyable. These individuals, at every stage of their careers, thought big and envisioned success. While the when and where of their corner office may have been unclear, the vivid and unwavering vision of making it happen was never a question. And once this image was created, their vocabulary and actions aligned in support of this goal.

John Eliot (2004) said, "Instead of limiting themselves to what's probable, the best performers will pursue the heart-pounding, exciting, really big, difference-making dreams" (p. xix). The same is true for these corner office executives, who bravely envisioned success in new and unique ways. P. K. Scheerle said it well: "If you are going to devote yourself to something, take bold action, do it big, and don't be afraid to stand alone."

We were quite surprised at the similarities in the executives' stories, and many used the same words in describing their journey to the corner office: "resilience," "focus on the future," "be bold in decision-making," "dissatisfaction with incremental change," "the need to be innovative," and "surround yourself with the best people and empower them," to name a few. Their stories provide a rich complement to the management literature, and we believe this is just the beginning of understanding what it takes for an executive nurse to achieve success in the corner office. We hope that this is simply the start of our dialogue around the new frontier for executive nurses. You, too, have the ability to aspire to the corner office, and we wish you success and fun as you begin your journey.

"Confidence is not a guarantee of success, but a pattern of thinking that will improve your likelihood of success."

–John Eliot

Executive Leadership Lessons

- From early in their student and professional lives, these executives deliberately managed their careers, seeking out the education and varied experiences that provided the foundation for positions of increasing scope and responsibility.

- Successful nurse executives do not see failure as failure—they view what others might consider to be failures as learning opportunities and take a very pragmatic approach: Assess the situation, understand the alternatives, mitigate the risk involved, and create opportunity where disappointment seems the likely outcome.

- A CEO or COO provides better informed leadership, makes smarter financial decisions, and negotiates better deals with key stakeholders after having benefited from deep understanding of all of the organization's critical functions.

- As rising stars within nursing are identified, health care leaders must consider the need to expose these up-and-comers to experiences outside of their discipline.

- As nurses rise within the executive ranks, they will be faced with an increasing demand for results and the need to fully understand the financial impacts on their organizations.

- The commonalities among successful nursing executives are striking and outline a clear path for others to follow.

References

Cohen, S. (2009). *Linking coaching to business results.* Right Management.

Dvorsky, G. (2012, July 16). Have we broken Olympic records for the last time? *Yahoo! Sports.* Retrieved from http://io9.com/5926368/have-we-broken-olympic-records-for-the-last-time

Eliot, J. (2004). *Overachievement: The new science of working less to accomplish more.* New York, NY: The Penguin Group.

Glassman, G. (n.d.). *What is CrossFit?* Retrieved from http://community.crossfit.com/what-is-crossfit

Hunt, J. M., & Weintraub, J. R. (2011). *The coaching manager: Developing top talent in business.* Thousand Oaks, CA: Sage Publications.

Institute of Medicine (IOM). (2010). *The future of nursing: Leading change, advancing health.* Washington, DC: The National Academies Press.

Lemanski, T. (n.d.). *Chicago executive coaching: Values and beliefs.* Retrieved from http://chicagoexecutivecoaching.com/executive-coaching-values-beliefs.htm

Michelman, P. (2004). Methodology: Do you need an executive coach? *Harvard Management Update, 9*(12).

Rosales, P. (2012). World record breakers at the 2012 Olympics. *Yahoo! Sports.* Retrieved from http://sports.yahoo.com/photos/ olympics-record-breakers-of-2012-1344773931-slideshow/

Silver, N. (2012, July 28). Which records get shattered? *The New York Times,* p. SR4.

Index